THE MYSTERY

OF

HUMAN AGING

THE MYSTERY

OF

HUMAN AGING

THE SURPRISING INSIGHTS OF
A SCIENCE THAT'S STILL YOUNG

BJÖRN SCHUMACHER

Translated from German
by Lyn Sengstacken

Algora Publishing
New York

Original title: Das Geheimnis des menschlichen Alterns. Die überraschenden
    Erkenntnisse der noch jungen Alternsforschung. By Björn Schumacher.
© 2015 by Karl Blessing Verlag, a division of Verlagsgruppe Random House GmbH,
München, Germany.

Library of Congress Cataloging-in-Publication Data —

Names: Schumacher, Björn, author.
Title: The mystery of human aging : the surprising insights of a science
    that's still young / Prof. Dr. Björn Schumacher.
Other titles: Geheimnis des menschlichen Alterns. English
Description: New York : Algora Publishing, [2017] | Includes bibliographical
    references and index.
Identifiers: LCCN 2017001192| ISBN 9781628942835 (hard cover : alk. paper) |
    ISBN 9781628942828 (soft cover : alk. paper) | ISBN 9781628942842 (pdf)
Subjects: | MESH: Aging
Classification: LCC QP86 | NLM WT 104 | DDC 612.6/7—dc23 LC record available at
https://lccn.loc.gov/2017001192

Printed in the United States

Dedicated to Pauline

TABLE OF CONTENTS

Foreword

By Prof. Dr. Jan Vijg

Aging is a problem that consumes us, literally and figuratively. Recent scientific insights into the process of age-related degeneration and death suggest new hopes for the future, but the problems have gripped humankind from the beginning.

From Antiquity to today, old age has generally been considered to begin around age 60. I was reminded of this recently when — at 62 — I automatically got a senior discount when buying a ticket for an art show in Manhattan (I didn't feel quite so bad after I was told that such discounts actually begin at 55 or 60).

To learn how others have dealt with old age, the best era we can compare ourselves with is the Roman Empire, about two millennia ago. While our own times are prosperous and seem optimally suited to produce a very large number of healthy elderly people, the citizens of the Roman Empire were perhaps even better off; Western Europe (which had been part of the Empire) only began to match Rome in the 18th century, with the beginning of the industrial revolution. The Roman Empire was a huge free-trade area — kept safe by a professional army counting one million men — that stretched from Scotland to Iraq and Romania to North Africa. And its wealth and stability did indeed allow many people to age well and long. But there are differences.

This is clear from writings from those days, most notably the letters from Pliny the Younger (A.D. c 61–113). Pliny wrote about some of the negative aspects of aging, and notes that one of his friends, Corellius Rufus, took his own life at age 67 because he was no longer able to bear the agony of disease. This sounds very familiar to us; in spite of the great progress in medical research over the last centuries, we are still confronted with the ravages of old age in exactly the same way.

Pliny was a member of the upper class. However, even most of his peers who died naturally were in their 60s or 70s, and sometimes 80s, but rarely beyond. Pliny himself died peacefully when he was 52. In Roman times, even for the very rich, almost nobody got past the age of 80.

The average person's life expectancy at birth has improved dramatically. About 2000 years ago, life expectancy at birth was not much higher than 25, mostly due to a high rate of child mortality. Nowadays this is much less of a problem and life expectancy at birth in the US is close to 80 years. The improvements in the human condition that led to these dramatic increases in healthy life span began in Europe in the late 18th century and were entirely due to one thing: science.

Science as we know it began in Europe in the 17th century, reaching high points in the 19th and 20th centuries. It is science that allowed the improvements in agriculture that gradually began to prevent famine. It is science that gave us an understanding of the germ theory of disease leading to preventative measures against infectious disease, from clean water to vaccination and antibiotics. It is science that was instrumental in understanding the risk factors for heart disease, and it was science that gave us the understanding as to how cancer originates, insights that now begin to reduce mortality for that disease. Now researchers are exploring whether science can also cure aging and extend our life span!

This is why *The Mystery of Human Aging — The Surprising Insights of A Science That's Still Young* by Björn Schumacher is so welcome. What is the nature of aging? Can science truly do something about it? What are its mechanisms? How does it relate to evolution? As the author says in the book, "To be able to defeat diseases, one must understand them," and nothing could be more true.

Schumacher's timing is impeccable. Because of the improvements in medical technology and increased access to medical care, a newborn's chances of surviving until a ripe old age have never been greater. This is good, but it also places an enormous strain on society to support the large numbers of aging baby boomers as they become eligible for social security and Medicare.

Schumacher describes these developments in detail. However, what he also does is to describe our options in terms of scientific developments that now, for the first time in history, allow us to understand the complicated biological processes that underlie aging.

Excitingly, this great understanding may one day lead to interventions to ward off the diseases of old age and, possibly, substantially increase our healthy life span.

In a tour de force the author explains in clear terms and for a broad audience what we know about the molecular, cellular and physiological basis of aging. He is able to do that because of his background in studying the molecular processes of aging himself in the laboratory. In his studies he uncovered some intriguing parallels between increased damage to DNA and the normal aging process: similar molecular pathways respond to aging and genotoxic stress in an attempt to survive. Such an evolutionarily conserved survival response now offers us many promising targets to develop novel therapies for aging-related diseases and, possibly, to delay aging itself.

After studying biology at the University of Constance, Germany, and the University of Stony Brook, NY, the author received his PhD training at the Max Planck Institute for Biochemistry in Martinsried, Germany. I first met Björn when he was a postdoctoral fellow in the laboratory of my collaborator Dr. Jan Hoeijmakers in Rotterdam, The Netherlands, now more than a decade ago. It was there where he performed the research that led to the discovery of the DNA damage-induced survival pathways that now offers us hope for developing anti-aging therapies. And I am proud to say that Björn's work was part of the large international project supported by the US National Institutes of Health, led by me, that is studying the possible role of damage to DNA as a cause of aging. Both Björn and I, therefore, are experts in this particular part of aging research.

However, both of us are also quick to broaden our interest into the realms of other disciplines if that gives us the opportunity to better understand what aging is and what our prospects are to successfully intervene in the process. Björn has been exceptionally successful in that endeavor.

He is now leading the Institute for Genome Stability in Aging and Disease at the University of Cologne in Germany and is one of the world's renowned experts in the biology of aging. It was in Cologne where he conceived of this book, and he must have spent many hours, days, weeks and months in trying to mold so many basic science concepts into a format accessible to a broad audience and still at a sufficiently high level to be of interest to his peers. In that he has succeeded magnificently!

In *The Mystery of Human Aging*, Björn takes you by the hand and guides you through a wondrous world of the accomplishments of biomedical research through the ages. You learn about the evolutionary origin of aging, the structure and function of DNA and how damage to that molecule can cause premature aging, but also about mitochondria, the cellular invaders that turned into our energy providers and are now suspected to be a major target of aging. He shows how the tiny nematode worm has been used to demonstrate, for the first time, that it is possible to extend the life span of a living organism by tinkering with its genes. You will learn about dietary restriction as a way to extend the healthy life span of many organisms, from the unicellular yeast to mice and rats, about the new drugs that now appear to do the same thing, and about the first hesitant attempts to begin the long road towards life extension in humans.

That last part, life extension in humans, gets ample attention in the book. It is pointed out that our genetic makeup, like that of most other organisms, is such that the genetic priority is to reproduce, not to preserve our body for an extended period after that reproductive phase. This may be hard to swallow, but our bodies were never designed for eternity, and immortality is not achievable. Instead, it is argued — and I fully agree — that our attention should be focused on extending the quality of life as long as possible.

In this respect, the author provides a wealth of examples as to how we can avoid many an age-related ailment simply by living healthily. We also learn about progress in curing diseases, such as cancer and Alzheimer's disease, both typically age-related diseases that have a much better chance of successful treatment when it is realized that both have their roots in the aging process. And we read about stem cell therapy and some newly-discovered proteins in blood from young individuals that can promote functional regeneration of aged stem cells.

Finally, the author discusses the impact of all this research, which started in the 19th century with the prevention of infectious disease, on an aging society. We learn about the demographic shifts which now give our economists headaches and the need to adapt to new circumstances. The book ends, most appropriately, with a plea for continuing knowledge gathering about who we are as humans and defining us in ever greater detail across our life span.

In summary, I strongly recommend *The Mystery of Human Aging* to those who want to know why and how they age. This is not a book for those who merely want to hear soothing stories about a future of immortality and science fiction. Instead, it is an essential resource for those truly interested in the science that for the first time in history enables us to understand what aging is all about, what the realistic future prospects are for further extending the healthy human life span and how society needs to adapt to the greatly altered demographics that result from this magnificent human endeavor of knowledge gathering. As such it is a must-read for anyone interested in the future of our aging society in America and elsewhere.

Jan Vijg, Ph.D.
Professor and Chair, Department of Genetics
Albert Einstein College of Medicine, New York,
www.einstein.yu.edu
Author of the books *Aging of the Genome* (Oxford
University Press, 2007) and
*The American Technological Challenge: Stagnation and
Decline in the 21st Century* (Algora, 2011)

Why Should I Read a Book About Aging Now?

Do you remember the first time? When you first realized that your life will come to an end? That your existence is fleeting and you're going to die? Perhaps this realization didn't strike you suddenly but dawned on you gradually. Often we become aware of the inevitability of death only when someone close to us dies. We feel how transitory our own life is when someone else passes away. Rare moments like these, when we stop and reflect, force us to reconsider the basics.

How do you think you will meet your end? How was it for your parents or grandparents? A sudden heart attack? Long suffering after a stroke? The slow progression of age-related dementia? Cancer, possibly with long and debilitating therapy? Or maybe an accident? Did they fade away in their sleep? Do you think about it? About the end, your end? Maybe you don't, at least not too often. It's hard to get on with living if you're caught up in thinking about death. You're not alone, here. Everyone knows that he will die. It doesn't take any particular intelligence or talent; we all know it. But we hardly ever talk about it.

And awareness of our own (impending) death is not new. Our ancestors figured out long ago that their existence was finite. We don't know when it first occurred to people that their existence was, in principle, limited; after all, our ancestors would have had to put it in writing, if they wanted to leave a record for posterity. And what could have been so important to the first literate people that they would put it in writing? Of course, trade and barter deals. They were concerned about increasing their wealth. Then, how about humankind's first epic poem? You guessed it; it's about the desire for immortality! You are clearly not the first person to think about his death. On the contrary, awareness of our own death is perhaps one of the first signs of human consciousness.

What has changed, since *Homo sapiens* — or maybe already a distant forefather — first recognized that existence was transient? The name "Homo sapiens" (literally "wise person capable of reflection") would truly be suitable for one who could come to such knowledge. And die we do, like any other living thing. Do we know more about it than our ancestors did? What would we tell them? We could go on talking day and night about the development of humanity, from religion and science to wars and world empires, philosophy and literature, technology and industry, illnesses and cures — but our mortality? Maybe we would just shrug and tell them, forget about it, that won't change in ten thousand, or a hundred thousand years.

Forgetting about it: that is, in fact, the way we usually manage to ignore our mortality. Even more, we repress all thought of it. Indeed, it is important that we repress it. People created many religions that, today, we may be rather inclined to smile at; and others which perhaps we can even sympathize with. The notion of a paradise to come was a perfect solution to the problem of death: there is life after death! Another solution, perhaps more plausible to some, was reincarnation on earth. A limited existence on earth doesn't seem so bad, as long as it goes on afterwards in the same or in a different form.

Life seems to get shorter towards the end, and it always ends in death. One could describe aging the same way. What do we know about aging? Aging is actually easier to grasp than death. If we cannot tell our prehistoric ancestors anything about a life after death, can we at least say something about aging? What is aging, how does it work, and why must we all age?

After reading this book, you will have something to tell them, because in fact our generation is the first in all the long history of humanity that has achieved any fundamental insights into the mystery of human aging. In recent years, there has been a veritable explosion of new knowledge about aging. And that is what this book is about.

I. Why Do We Age? A Question as Old as Humankind

I.1. What is aging?

First of all, let's define aging — something we do every second of our lives. Then we'll learn why living and aging are inseparable and why, for better or worse, we can never be like Dorian Gray. But rather than learning from a hundred-year-old that cigarettes don't do any harm, you will meet a pair of fraternal twins: chronological and biological age.

Perhaps the most amazing feature of human culture is that we are conscious of ourselves, of our aging and our death. We are all aging, every year, every day, every minute of our lives. There is no exception, no delay. Some people age faster, some slower. One man will be decrepit at seventy while another man — or more often another woman — at ninety. On average, women live longer than men. However, precisely because they live longer, women suffer more from diseases in old age.

What is aging? The term aging is commonly defined as the gradual reduction of the efficiency of the organs, tissues and cells, while at the same time the probability of falling ill and dying increases. Interestingly, we have no word for an increase in the number of passing years of life without aging, such as what happened to Dorian Gray, whose portrait aged in his place. There is no getting old without "aging," not even as a linguistic concept. Humankind cannot get older without aging. Our life is therefore characterized by aging; life and aging cannot be separated.

There are different views on when aging begins. The ancient Greeks considered the high point of life to be the early twenties, and in fact there is some evidence that the gradual dismantling, the degeneration, begins in the mid-twenties. It might also be said that aging begins as soon as our physical development and growth are complete. However, it's not so easy to define that point, because different organs become fully formed at different stages in the development of the human body.

We recognize the signs of aging quite readily, albeit perhaps not so quickly in ourselves as in others. People can often make a reasonably good estimate of another person's age just by looking at the face — at least, if cosmetic surgery and botox injections have not been used to disguise the outer signs of aging. Certainly there are differences between "biological" age and "chronological" age. Being able to recognize and measure the different aspects of human aging is of great importance for the medical field.

Chronological age is merely our age since we have been born and states how long we've been alive; that's something that can be known exactly in almost everyone's case. But when it is not known, it can be quite a challenge to determine one's chronological age — for example for forensic doctors, in criminal cases, when someone's identity papers have been lost or falsified. To determine someone's biological age is anything but trivial; it is not at all the same as chronological age, especially in the later years of life.

Biological age shows where you are within your own individual life span and how many more years you can look forward to. Some people enjoy an exceptionally long life. The Frenchwoman Jeanne Calment was a record breaker in this respect. She died in 1997 at the age of one hundred and twenty-two years — just three years after she quit smoking, and that, only because her progressive blindness made it too hard for her to light her own cigarettes. Being dependent on others even for lighting a cigarette was no option for this strong-willed lady. Jeanne Calment and other centenarians aged, biologically, extremely slowly. In a later chapter we will look at people who, on the contrary, age so rapidly that even as children they already resemble the elderly.

Measuring biological aging is especially important if you want to know whether the aging process can be delayed or if you are subject to the influences of accelerated aging. Currently, huge numbers of researchers and physicians around the world are investigating how we can measure biological age. No reliable "biomarkers" of aging have been identified so far, although there are some promising candidates. The problem of finding such a biomarker is that people age very differently. One may have a very high risk of heart attack, while another suffers kidney or liver failure. Not every organ ages at the same speed in each one of us. Also, we are each somewhat different when it comes to outward signs of aging; some people have a full head of gray hair while others start going bald by the age of thirty. This is partly due to the fact that every person is born with a very individual genetic composition. The only exceptions are identical twins. But even they, like all of us, experience very different environmental influences and stressors during the course of their lives. No one person is exactly the same as another; each of us is unique.

Currently, it is assumed that by combining a sufficient number of biomarkers we should be able to make a relatively good prediction of a human being's biological age. Without the development of such reliable biomarkers of age, it is nearly impossible to find ways to intervene — as we will discuss in the final chapter. Finally, you can only determine ten, twenty or more years later whether a treatment has had a positive effect or you should have tried something else. Just to determine the biological age is, in itself, a challenge. The question of human aging presents us with many puzzles, and the detective work of the investigation is in full swing.

I.2. Aging and death in the earliest written testimonies

Apparently there is no medicinal plant that can prevent death — even if Gilgamesh is said to have picked one! In the next section you will find out why people have been seeking to avoid death for thousands of years but are still dying, nonetheless. The following appear as witnesses of this human failure: Qin Shihuangdi, Ramses II, Methuselah and Hippocrates, and even Cleopatra, who sought to drown death in warm mare's milk.

To achieve a ripe old age has indeed been desirable since time immemorial, and still today (in some cultures, at least) older people are met with particular respect. Already in antiquity, there were people who achieved a very advanced age. It is reported that the pharaoh Ramses II not only begat surprisingly many children — nearly a hundred daughters and sons are attributed to him — but also that he was almost ninety years old when he died. The biblical story of Methuselah, who is supposed to have begotten Lemach at the age of 187 (Genesis 5:25), also suggests that long before modern medicine and our present lifestyle with its emphasis on healthy practices, some people lived to a remarkably old age. Advanced age, however, was a rare privilege.

Only in the last two centuries has the average life expectancy risen dramatically. Until then, a life expectancy in the mid-thirties was normal. This low life expectancy was in part attributable to the high infant mortality rate — at the beginning of the Industrial Revolution almost one in every four children died. Those who survived childhood enjoyed a life span of just over forty years on average. Infectious diseases were especially devastating. There were no vaccines or antibiotics; diseases plagued cities, and there were chronic food shortages, especially among the poor rural population, such as we can no longer imagine today in our latitudes. Just by pushing back child mortality through modern civilizational achievements, above all medicine, we have steadily increased life expectancy. Of course, adults also benefit from advances in medicine and hygiene, better nutrition, and lifestyle improvements.

Although the topic of aging has pre-occupied humankind for several thousand years, no one knew why we age, and above all what factors drive the process of aging. Immortality was already the theme of what may be the oldest epic of humanity, *The Epic of Gilgamesh* [1]. The story probably dates to the third millennium before our era; it was put in writing by the beginning of the second millennium BC. The epos was handed down to us, chiseled on twelve clay tablets, kiln fired, that thus survived the millennia. Gilgamesh, two-thirds god, one-third human, was the king of Uruk, one of the first human cities, located in Mesopotamia, the "land between the Euphrates and the Tigris." The ruins of the city of Uruk are in today's Iraq. The people of Uruk suffered under their despotic sovereign who imposed immense burdens on them; they were exhausted and begged the gods for help. They sent the man-beast Enkido to challenge the king. However, after having been civilized by cohabiting with a temple priestess, Enkido instead turned to become Gilgamesh's close friend. Together the friends went through many adventures, until Gilgamesh spurned the love of the city's goddess of protection, and the rejected lover avenged herself by causing Enkido to fall sick and die. Through the loss of his friend, Gilgamesh came to face his own mortality and began to fear death.

On a trip similar to Homer's Odyssey, he sought out the wise man Utnapishtim. (The original model for the biblical Noah, he survived the great flood when the gods decided that humanity had to be decimated; and now an infinitely long life on the edge of the earth resulted.) But Utnapishtim was reluctant to open up to Gilgamesh. The king was required to stay awake for seven days continuously in order to achieve immortality. However — exhausted from his journey to the edge of the world — he fell into a sleep of just that duration, and so he remained mortal. Then there was a plant to be plucked from the bottom of the sea, which is also referred to as the elixir of immortality. After Gilgamesh accomplished this feat, a snake stole the herb of immortality from him while he was napping. The beast then began, by continuously shedding its skin, an endless life. The great King Gilgamesh eventually recognized that the desire for immortality was in vain and he would share the fate that his friend Enkido had suffered.

The life of the first Emperor of China, Qin Shihuangdi, was similarly marked by the fear of his own death. A fierce ruler in the third century BC, he subdued all the other kingdoms of China through his military superiority, but he was constantly exposed to assassination attempts. He feared death. Seeking an "Isle of the Immortal," he sent out his fleet, but it never returned — perhaps the sailors were afraid what fate would await them if they should come back without the elixir of immortality. Out of fear of his own death, the emperor now turned to various healers. They promised to save his life by dosing him with mercury. No one suspected at that time that mercury is highly toxic. Qin probably died of mercury poisoning; so he was a victim of his own urge for immortality. Only hope is eternal: Qin left a whole army of life-sized terracotta warriors in his burial chamber to protect him ever after, and one may visit them even today near the central Chinese city of Xi'an.

And death is not all that people seek to defy. The quest for eternal youth has been prevalent throughout the history of humanity since ancient times. The ancient Egyptians are generally regarded as the inventors of cosmetics; evidence of their pioneering medical treatments has also survived. Cleopatra is said to have bathed daily in honey and milk to maintain her youthful pharaonic complexion — and the lust of Roman rulers. From Hippocrates — the "father of medicine" — to Galen, the famous healers of antiquity learned their craft in Egypt. The ancient Egyptians had many cosmetic and medicinal formulas.

The Greeks were particularly aware of the crux of the problem inherent in immortality, as Greek mythology testifies. The goddess Eos loved the mortal Tithonos with an undying love, in the truest sense of the word "undying." She asked Zeus to grant Tithonos immortality, but — perhaps blinded by love — she forgot that Tithonos would age. So he was fated to live on and on, long after his youthful charms faded and the infirmities of age were all too apparent. The picture of Eos and Tithonos foreshadowed the terrible scenario before our eyes today, the fate that threatens an aging society: getting older and older, more and more decrepit, without death to draw things to a close.

For millennia humankind has desperately fought aging and death, seeking magic potions and a Fountain of Youth, but nothing has changed our inevitable fate. And while our knowledge of life has been revolutionized by the biological research of the last two centuries, the molecular mechanisms of aging have only begun to become clear in the last two decades.

What do we know today about aging? Will we be able to prevent many age-related diseases in the future? Since aging is a biological process, we'll begin with some basic considerations of biological evolution. In biology, it is of paramount importance to see every process in the context of the history of evolution. Only in this way can we achieve a real understanding of aging.

Next, we'll look at those genes that are of particular importance for aging. Some people carry defective genes that accelerate the aging process.

Others enjoy unusually long lives thanks to their genetic structure. The understanding of the genetics of aging is thus particularly important.

Add in the environmental influences, which can have a positive or negative influence on life expectancy. Understanding these mechanisms offers the prospect of modern biomedical research finding new therapies to prevent age-related diseases.

Finally, I will discuss the profound changes in the shifting age structure, which our society will have to respond to. Today we are at an important crossroads. The aging of society could lead us into the abyss of morbidity, but it also could offer many people opportunities for a longer and better life. We have our future in our hands, for never before did humankind know more about itself, its aging process and its illnesses.

I.3. The origin of aging and the building blocks of life

Now, we'll have a report on the birth of life (Time: the darkest past; Location: the primordial atmosphere; Producer: DNA, RNA, amino acids), and on its development and the language that it learned over millions of years (ATGC).

We'll also hear about the birth of Molecular Biology, which is dedicated to the exploration of life (Time: the 1930s; Location: Cold Spring Harbor, NY; Producers: Biology, with Physics and Chemistry assisting).

We'll meet the people — and the kitchen mixer — that have been instrumental to the solution of various puzzles: the scientists who brewed phagocyte cocktails and the agnostics who spelled out the theories.

A life without aging seems inconceivable; aging is the natural consequence of living. Why is this link so inexorable? Why is aging an inherent property of life? Looking more closely at how aging occurs throughout our body, there is one fundamental exception: our "seed" remains immortal. Again and again, in every generation for millions of years, the fusion of the egg and sperm have set the biological clock back to zero. The continuation of life is so all-encompassing that all life on earth can be traced back to a common primitive life form, originating somewhere in the primordial soup. As Rudolf Virchow stated: "Omnis cellula e cellula" — a cell can only emerge from a cell. All living beings, whether human, monkey, dog, worm, plant, mushroom, or yes, even bacteria that were formed four billion years ago in an original atmosphere — had a single common ancestor.

The prerequisite for the emergence of life was, first of all, the formation of organic matter in the atmosphere. Initially there were only inorganic gases such as carbon dioxide, nitrogen and hydrogen sulfide. Life as we know it, however, is based on organic matter, which can form more complex molecules. Organic matter is built on carbon that is compounded with other carbon atoms as well as with hydrogen, oxygen, nitrogen and other elements. The propensity of carbon to form many bonds allows the formation of macromolecules, far larger structures, which take different forms and can even perform functions, like molecular machines.

How could organic substances be produced from the gases of the primordial atmosphere, when the earth was young? Stanley Miller and Harold Urey conducted a key experiment in the 1950s at the University of Chicago that casts light on the dark past [2]. These two American scientists created sealed vials containing the elements that were, at that time, thought to reflect the contents of earth's early atmosphere. In order to inject energy into their experimental system, swirling with these inorganic gases, they sparked it with an electrical charge — emulating the lightning that is believed to have been present in Earth's early atmosphere. What Miller and Urey obtained in this way was, in fact, the chemical origin of life: from these gases they synthesized amino acids, and similar experiments that followed yielded the bases of deoxyribonucleic acid (DNA) and ribonucleic acid (RNA). DNA, RNA, and amino acids: These are the chemical building blocks of life, from bacteria all the way to humans.[1]

During the next decade it was discovered that DNA and RNA function as the carrier or transferee of information by which proteins are built from amino acids. Miller and Urey had the proof that the basic building blocks of life could come from the original atmosphere.

Another prerequisite that was absolutely essential for life was reproduction, i.e., the ability of a structure to restore or replicate itself. Otherwise the formation of a structure would only be a very temporary event, and through the inevitable damage — one can imagine the inhospitable conditions of the early atmosphere — this structure would very quickly be lost again. Here, the enzymatic activity of RNA plays a critical role: apart from its role as a repository of information RNA can copy and thus reproduce itself. And this is why RNA is considered to have been the basis for life 4 billion years ago. Only later, once proteins became available as the main enzymes for copying, did the chemically more stable DNA replace RNA as the carrier of genetic information. DNA can carry much more genetic information than RNA and, through an endless process of copy and change, spread biological life further. DNA is the genetic basis of all animals, plants, fungi, bacteria and even many viruses.

DNA consists of long chains of a sequence of four *nucleotides*: the *bases*, adenine, thymine, guanine and cytosine (ATGC for short) — each with a sugar, *ribose* — all connected by a *phosphate chain* as a backbone.

---

1 It is now assumed that the first organic substances from which life originated came from hydrothermal vents in the sea floor, that is, underwater geysers or "white smokers."

ATGC is the language in which life is encoded. The sequence of these four bases determines how the Flagellum, the filamentary, moving structure on the surface of a bacterium, works; how a plant takes in the energy of sunlight; how our brain and heart are formed; how we breathe, or run — and how we age.

The nucleotides are connected in long chains to form strands of DNA. Two individual strands combine into a double helix, through which the pairs of bases are held together. An A is always paired with a T, and a G with a C.

Alfred Hershey and Martha Chase set out to prove that DNA contains genetic information, in their laboratory in the idyllic Cold Spring Harbor on Long Island, just about an hour outside of New York City, in the early 1950s[3]. The Cold Spring Harbor Laboratory had become the birthplace of a completely new branch of biology, *molecular biology*, in the late 1930s.

The science journalist Horace Judson describes the beginnings of molecular Biology in his wonderful work *The Eighth Day of Creation* [4]. Every summer the pioneers of this new discipline met to exchange their latest ideas. Molecular Biology sought to understand life, starting with its smallest, most basic structures. This was a completely new approach, because biology at the time was not a particularly mechanistic discipline. Only in the mid-1940s did physicists begin to take an interest in the functioning of life, and this gave biology a completely new impetus. At that time there were many physicists, like the brilliant theorist Leo Szilard, who looked back with indignation and horror at the role they themselves had played in the "Manhattan Project" for the development of the atomic bomb which had been used to wreak such terrible suffering on Hiroshima and Nagasaki. These morally responsible researchers wanted to dedicate their lives henceforth to using physics for positive and life-affirming purposes.

Until that time, biology had been a mostly descriptive science. Botanists, zoologists, and embryologists made observations of living things in order to advance our understanding of nature. Physicists and scientists from other disciplines as well, such as chemistry, became increasingly interested in biology and they began to quantify, i.e., to measure, how biology operates.

Bacteriophages turned out to play a special role in this. Small viruses that infect bacteria, bacteriophages are very similar to the viruses that are such a scourge to us humans. They attach themselves to the surface of bacteria and deposit their genetic material in each infected bacterium. This leaves the bacteriophage living on the surface of the bacteria. It's not long before the bacterium is converted into a bacteriophage production plant — until it bursts, and plenty of new bacteriophages are released.

One morning, Alfred Hershey asked his wife to let him use the kitchen mixer in the laboratory. He poured some bacteriophage-infected bacteria into the mixer and turned it on, so that the docked bacteriophage covers were thrown off the bacteria. Prior to infection, Hershey and Chase had marked the bacteriophages with radioactive sulfur, and in a second test marked them with radioactive phosphate. While the sulfur could only mark the proteins, the phosphate actually marked the DNA of the bacteriophages. After shaking off the bacteriophage from the cell walls in the mixer, the researchers separated the heavy bacteria from the lighter bacteriophage covers by running them through a centrifuge. The radioactive sulfur was then found exclusively in the batch containing the bacteriophage covers, while the radioactive phosphate was in the bacteria. From these bacteria, which contained only bacteriophage DNA but no original bacteriophage protein, new phages were produced. This was proof that genetic information is encoded and transmitted in the DNA, not in the proteins.

The structure of DNA and thus the structure of genes were revealed just a short time later by James Watson and Francis Crick. James Watson, who as a student had already attended a summer course in Cold Spring Harbor, visited Cambridge, England, and worked together with the perceptive physicist Francis Crick. Both wanted to find out what our genetic material and DNA looked like.

This required getting a picture of DNA. Images of tiny structures such as DNA could be acquired using x-ray crystallography. However, this was no easy task. First of all, you need to get the molecule, in this case DNA, in crystal form. Then an x-ray was taken which allowed them to map the varied shadings of the crystal. Now that they had acquired a usable picture of the crystal, the actual work began: from this point, they had to "interpret" the shadings to derive an actual idea of the form. Watson and Crick were an excellent team: the British physicist could perform the calculations based on the x-ray structure, while the American from Chicago rolled up his sleeves and tinkered about with cardboard, constructing possible models of DNA. First, they needed that x-ray image of DNA. Watson managed to get a picture from a biochemist specializing in x-ray structure analysis, Rosalind Franklin.

In hindsight there has been considerable speculation as to how Watson arrived at this image and why Franklin had not figured out the structure of DNA herself. Franklin had worked a long time on interpreting her DNA x-ray images. She might have considered too limited a range of alternatives for deriving the structure, while the intellectual duo of Watson & Crick played with the craziest ideas every day. According to Watson, who in the course of his long life wrote some books about this period that make for very interesting reading, Franklin was no longer interested in DNA and therefore willingly let him use her footage.

The discovery of the double helix structure of DNA must be one of the greatest scientific breakthroughs ever. Watson and Crick published their results in 1953, describing the mechanism by which DNA is copied and thus how life is reproduced [5]. Now people could picture pretty well how the double helix of DNA divides and how an older strand serves as a template for a new copy of the DNA. With each cell division, an older strand of DNA is used as template for the synthesis of a new strand to form two daughter cells.

Watson went on to teach at Harvard University while Crick began working intensively to study how the information of the DNA could be transmitted in the formation of proteins. Crick formulated the "central dogma" of molecular biology. According to this idea, the information flows from the DNA to the RNA to the proteins, which consist of sequences of amino acids. Through the various properties of the amino acids, the proteins can take very different forms and perform very different functions; they can form a variety of structures or serve as enzymes that catalyze chemical reactions.

Later, the passionate agnostic Crick once said that he used the word "dogma" because, in his view, that religious term was the correct way to label a claim for which no one had the slightest evidence. But Crick was correct in his central dogma [6]. DNA is first transcribed into RNA. The term *transcription* is derived from the Latin *trans scribere* — to write over again. Here, it refers to the process by which the details of hereditary information, i.e., the DNA, are transcribed to form copies of RNA chains. In this way information is transferred through RNA copies into proteins. RNA molecules are almost identical to DNA strand except for thymine, which in RNA is replaced by uracil. The RNA chain can be transported out of the cell nucleus and then translated into protein. The RNA is a "messenger" between the DNA and proteins, and it is therefore also called mRNA. By using the mRNA, the DNA can stay in the cell nucleus forever. Through this translation, the sequence of the RNA bases is then converted into a sequence of amino acids, that is, the structure of proteins: *protein biosynthesis*.

Proteins may consist of short or long chains, formed by very different sequences of twenty different amino acids. Proteins can be quite small, when only a few amino acids form a *peptide*, or they can build huge structures such as muscle fibers. During the course of protein biosynthesis, long chains of amino acids can make three-dimensional folds and thus may form highly complex structures.

Crick's central dogma has held up very well even to this day, although significant exceptions have been found. Nature is, in any event, far more diverse than any one rule can describe. RNA can even be transcribed in reverse into DNA. RNA can also be copied into RNA, for example when RNA viruses infect a cell. Even certain proteins, *prions* (well known from mad cow disease in the 1990s), can replicate themselves by folding other proteins into copies of themselves.

How can the sequence of four nucleotides determine the formation of proteins? Together with Sydney Brenner, a British scientist born in South Africa, Crick went on to formulate theories as to how the information contained in the sequence of the four nucleotides could be transferred in the formation of protein structures [7]. Crick and Brenner reasoned that cells would use the twenty most commonly found amino acids ignoring other less common amino acids. Now, if four nucleotides are supposed to determine all the possible sequences of twenty amino acids, of course one nucleotide cannot provide the coding of one amino acid, nor would two be enough. If they were only two bases in length, then only sixteen unique sequences could be made — there are only sixteen possible combinations — while there are twenty amino acids. A sequence of at least three nucleotides is needed to encode a given amino acid.

In addition, you need a signal to "start" and one to "stop." At this point Crick and Brenner still knew nothing about the complex mechanisms that regulate transcription and translation. So, first they came up with a very simple picture of transcription, in which a "comma-free" code precisely defines the amino acid sequence. In subsequent years of intensive experimental work on the "Language of Life," the DNA code, revealed that the reality is far less beautiful and far more complex than Crick and Brenner's ideas, even though they were right that the code is made up of triplets: The sequence of three nucleotides forms the codon by which an amino acid is encoded. Triple combinations could theoretically provide 64 amino acids, but only twenty are necessary. So there are several triplets of nucleotides coding for the different amino acids; and there is a "start" codon that specifies where the translation into amino acids begins and three stop codons that set the end of the chain of amino acids that create a protein. Regulating how and when genes are transcribed and translated into proteins has proven to be a very complex process that even today remains the subject of intense research.

I.4. Aging is an ancient property of life

Aging has a long tradition — it's been going on since our time as single-cell organisms!
You will now learn why a mother is always older than her daughter — even in yeast cells — and why not even symmetry could protect us against this fact.

Life could not last long if it were made up of isolated molecules like those of RNA or DNA alone, because these molecules were not very stable when exposed to the weather conditions of the primordial atmosphere. Therefore, it was important that fatty acids could form a closed system to protect the genetic material, the way droplets of fat float on water. Such a protective layer covers unicellular organisms and bacteria as well as all the cells — according to a recent estimate, 3.7×10^{13}, or 37 with twelve zeros — of the human body [8]. And it is not only the genetic information contained in the DNA molecules that needs to be reproduced but the whole cell and the entire contents of the cell.

In prokaryotes (from the Greek *pro* meaning "for," and *karyon*, "kernel" or "nut," that is, nucleus) such as bacteria, this is still a relatively simple process, in which all the molecules must be apportioned between the two daughter cells. In eukaryotes (*eu*, "real"), in other words all animals, plants and fungi, various cell compartments must also be parceled out. These cell compartments, technically *organelles*, allow the creation of specialized areas within a cell in which certain tasks can be carried out. Eukaryotes possess the nuclei (for which they are named), in which the genetic material is encapsulated and protected, the mitochondria responsible for the production of energy in the cells, and other organelles such as the Golgi apparatus, the endoplasmic reticulum, lysosomes and, in plants, the chloroplasts, which take the energy of sunlight and transform it to produce organic substances through photosynthesis.[1]

Through cell division, biological life expanded to cover the entire earth, from the depths of the sea to the peaks of the mountains. Before cell division can take place, the genetic material must be doubled so that each daughter cell can receive the full information. Even organelles and molecules must be distributed to the daughter cells. Through continual cell divisions a whole colony is created from one bacterium — and from one fertilized egg, an embryo and finally a whole human.

While the DNA strands are duplicated before the cell division takes place, other molecules can simply be divided — with the DNA, each cell inherits all the information needed to form all the other cell components. Thus each cell has both old molecules and new ones, just formed out of the information from the DNA.

For a long time it was assumed that unicellular organisms do not age because each cell divides in two, and it was believed that the contents of

---

1 Mitochondria and chloroplasts became part of the life of eukaryotes long ago and in an extraordinary way. The two types of organelles were originally bacteria that were "swallowed" at some point by eukaryotes and as *endosymbionts* (from Greek *endo* "inside" and *symbiosis*, "living together") and have now become inseparable parts of our cells.

the parent cell were divided evenly. Only recently was it recognized that the cell contents might be distributed differently between the two daughter cells. This was first observed in yeast cells by David Sinclair and Leonard Guarente, researchers in Boston. They were studying the different breakdown of small, specialized — and seemingly completely useless — circular pieces of DNA during the division of yeast cells. [1]

Baker's yeast is a single-cell fungus, and a mother cell will give rise to a new bud through cell division. The daughter cell may even live longer than the parent cell and generate a higher number of consecutive progeny. Thus the mother cell is "older" than the daughter cell. Sinclair and Guarente found that the small circular pieces of DNA accumulate in the mother cell and are not passed on to the daughter cell [9]. When, however, a protein known as *Sirtuin* prevented the formation of these small pieces of DNA, the mother cell could live longer.

Thomas Nyström, in Sweden, showed some years later that damaged proteins also remain in the mother cell while the daughter cell receives newer proteins and therefore stays "young" [10]. So it was clear that not only animals and plants, but even unicellular organisms, age.

In fact, Martin Ackermann and his colleagues discovered that even bacteria age. The bacterium *Caulobacter crescentus* is found in rivers and lakes and divides when an adhered mother cell produces a free-floating daughter cell, which then migrates to new realms. Ackermann observed the reproduction of the parent cell over three hundred hours and found that the mother cell would take longer and longer to generate a new cell, and sometimes reproduction would cease completely. Although it was long believed that aging was an invention of multi-cell organisms, the observations of Guarente, Sinclair, Nyström, Ackermann and their colleagues show that aging goes back to the origin of living organisms.

Baker's yeast and *C. crescentus* have in common that they divide *asymmetrically*, i.e., unequally. Many other unicellular organisms divide *symmetrically*; they grow apart and split in the middle. It is now assumed that aging comes into play when a mother and a daughter cell are formed, and asymmetry is the source of aging.

What is more, aging is already a factor in symmetric cell division; this was shown by Eric Stewart just a few years ago [11]. He filmed the cell division of *Escherichia coli*, a bacterium, which forms part of our natural intestinal flora. *E. coli* is probably the best-studied bacterium and it is indispensable to much laboratory work. The rod-shaped bacteria grow longitudinally into

---

1   These are pieces of ribosomal DNA (rDNA) encoding ribosomal RNA. Although rDNA is found in any genome, including the human, the formation of circular rDNA pieces cut from the genome appears to be a very specific feature of baker's yeast.

both poles and split in the middle. Stewart made a live film that tracked the daughter cells to see what would happen to those that inherited the "old" pole. Each time the cell divides, each of the new cells receives one old pole and forms a new pole where the center of the mother cell was. In the next cell division, one daughter cell gets the old pole and the other one gets the new pole, and so on and so on.

Stewart noted that when the descendants retained the old pole, fewer of them were able to reproduce and they died earlier than the cells that had received the new pole. So it became clear that aging was an ancient tradition in the history of life. It is also easy to demonstrate mathematically that with even a slight loss of function, for instance due to accumulated damage over time, it is beneficial to separate old and young components and by this means produce "rejuvenated" new cells that have an advantage for future growth.

I.5. The body ages, the germ line lives on

How and when did we learn to distinguish between somatic cells and germ cells? As soon as the germ line has been passed on, there is no need to preserve the body — this is the key to the evolutionary biology behind the mystery of aging. In fact, one cellular biologist in particular studied what limits the life of somatic cells (it is now called the "Hayflick limit").

While our body ages and dies, with each generation our germinal cells carry forward the transmission of our genes. With every oocyte, or egg fertilized by a sperm (also called a spermatozoon), the biological clock is set back to zero. When a new person is born, the germinal cells are the foundation of the next generation. Our germ line can theoretically go on to infinity, while the existence of the body ends.

The fundamental distinction between germ cells and ordinary somatic cells (or "body" cells; Greek *soma* = "body"), was first made by the renowned zoologist and evolutionary theorist August Weismann from Freiburg, Germany, toward the end of the 19th century. Weismann realized that there is a fundamental distinction between germ cells and somatic cells. Based on this distinction the body is arguably of no further use once the germ line has been renewed with each generation. Thus the evolutionary biologist explained the basic cause of aging: Preserving the body is clearly no longer necessary after successful procreation. The limited life span is therefore a fundamental property of the body.

The limited life span of the somatic cells was only proven experimentally in the early 1960s, when the cell biologist Leonard Hayflick was growing human somatic cells in a culture dish [12]. Cell growth in this context means that the cells propagate by division. Hayflick observed that the cells grew vigorously at first, multiplying themselves many times over, but then they invariably moved into a stationary phase and eventually stopped dividing. Ever since, this limitation of cell growth has been known as the "Hayflick limit," and the biological phenomenon is called *cellular senescence*, derived from the Latin word for "aging," *senescere*. We will look at cellular senescence later in a completely different context.

Weismann first assumed that the significance of aging is that it enables populations to clear themselves of frail individuals. He himself went on to revise his description of this "feature" of aging during his own lifetime, but he was heavily criticized for the statement nonetheless. The view that aging plays a positive role, indeed, is even necessary in order to make room for the young, is as widespread as it is false. The reasoning is circular: Humans age in order to make room for young people, but it's because they are old that they should yield to the young. In addition, one would have to invoke "group selection" that would weed out the group of older individuals because they are no longer necessary for the continued existence of the species. Group selection, however, doesn't work because as soon as one individual cheats and simply continues to live, that one would win against all the others and thus the entire property of aging would vanish from the species. Selection never takes place at the level of groups — not for aging or any other biological process.

Since life as it exists today was formed through evolutionary history, the following chapter will consider aging in conjunction with the theory of evolution: according to Theodosius Dobzhansky's famous dictum, "Nothing in biology makes sense except in the light of evolution"! Next, then, the effective forces of evolution will be explained as to how important biologists have recognized them.

I.6. Aging plays no role in evolution

First, Mr. Medawar explains what people and test tubes have in common. Then we'll learn what drives the aging process and how it is that we still enjoy the benefits of old age. Finally, Darwin helps us understand why evolution invests in our youth and why, after using the genetic material, our species seeks to compost the physical packaging it came in, as soon as possible.

That aging simply plays no role in evolution was elegantly proven by one of the most brilliant British researchers, the zoologist Peter Medawar,[1] in the

---

1 Interestingly, Medawar received the Nobel Prize for a whole other ground-breaking discovery during the Second World War when he was working — as it was customary for scientists in those times — in war-related medical research. He experimented on methods for transplanting skin in order to treat the burns of wounded British soldiers. In his work he showed that the rejection of tissues

1950s [13]. In order to demonstrate that aging is a passive biological property, Medawar chose to make a comparison with test tubes, which may break after a certain service life. For as long as the tubes are replaced frequently, it makes no difference if they last longer. They only need to hold up until they are replaced. The same applies to natural living things: what is decisive is survival at a young age, until offspring is begotten. How long an individual survives after reproducing is simply not important.

For a better understanding, here is a little excursion into the theory of evolution. Charles Darwin's theory is considered to be the biggest revolution in human thought, on a par with the Copernican revolution, which brought to light the fact that the earth is not at the center of the universe (and by extension neither are humans). Darwin, with his incredibly sharp powers of observation, travelled the world on board the *Beagle*. In doing so, he discovered that animals were not created entirely perfect, but in each case represent intermediate stages of development [14]. Darwin came to the conclusion that the species are not fixed or final creations but rather represent an intermediate product in an ongoing process of continual development and evolution, shaped by natural selection. Here, the concept of *fitness*, frequently misunderstood as "strongest," in fact means how "well adapted" an organism is to survive and procreate in its environment. Those who are best adapted to their environment are the ones who will survive. This is not necessarily the "strongest" but the one who can successfully reproduce.

Medawar placed aging in the context of the Darwinian theory of evolution. What is crucial to the concept of "fitness" is that the species continues to reproduce. A species is an evolutionary success if individuals are well enough adapted to produce offspring before the probability of dying is too high. Considering the many possible causes of death in the natural environment, it is readily apparent that an individual's resources are invested in survival during the early part of life, up to the age of reproduction. After successful reproduction, the pressure of selection is sharply reduced; the species is kept going by the younger generation.

Natural selection takes place at the level of the genes: the gene pool that is passed on successfully prevails in evolution. Consequently, Medawar realized, genes that contribute to fitness early in life are preserved in the gene pool of the species. By contrast, genes that reduce fitness in the early stages are selected out of the gene pool because the carriers of such genes have a lower probability of reproducing.

By the same token, there is no selection against those genes that exercise a negative impact only in later stages of life, after reproduction has taken

---

and organs upon transplantation was due to the recipient's immune system, an insight that even today is of paramount importance in transplantation medicine.

place. This is because the long-term survival of the parents is not necessary for the evolutionary success of the species. Such genes with later negative effects will remain in the gene pool; the process of selection is blind to them.

Based on these considerations, in the late 1970s the English biologist Thomas Kirkwood came up with the theory of *disposable soma*. This theory has gained considerable currency in modern gerontology. Kirkwood initially rediscovered August Weismann's writings on the problems of aging, and he recognized the full range of its implications [15]. He came to the conclusion that in the early phase of life, resources must be balanced between the preservation of bodily function and reproduction, in order to achieve the greatest success in transmission. After successful propagation, the somatic functions no longer need to be maintained and the individual's body may be disposed of, since it has no positive influence on further evolutionary success. In terms of evolution, conservation of bodily function after reproduction is useless, and that is the fundamental cause of frailty, illness and weakness in old age: Animals such as humans are not "fit" or not adapted to living long after they reproduce. Our genetic composition is not weeded and pruned to keep our bodies going forever.

I.7. Tracking down what makes aging inevitable

How can genes that have a positive effect while we're young turn out to be our downfall as we grow older? As we change (physically) over time, how do "free radicals" change the aging structures?

Building on the work of Peter Brian Medawar in the 1950s, American evolutionary biologist George Williams posited the concept of *antagonistic pleiotropy* as a cause of senescence. He used the Greek words *pleio* = "full" and *trop* = "rotation" or "turn" to describe the idea that genes have not only one but several different functions. Williams postulated that the same genes, which in our youthful years have positive effects, could, when we are older, play a negative role. This is an interesting idea that is still important nowadays in research on aging. It is particularly important because it presumes that aging is an inevitable consequence of living. In other words, aging is the price we pay for our vigor earlier in life.

The advanced ages we reach today were attained only very rarely in all our evolutionary history. Although there are quite a few examples of species having a particularly long life, in general animals face such a wide range of threats that only a very small part of the population can enjoy a long life. This also applied to earlier humans. They were exposed to many deadly infectious diseases. Then there were hunger and natural threats, and probably also the all-too-human occurrence of violence between peers. It is mainly due to medical progress and hygiene that we are largely exempt from such external threats today. The discovery of antibiotics and vaccines have transformed our life probably more than any other cultural achievement. So we more often enjoy the privilege of old age, which very few of our ancestors could dream of.

Damage to cell structures was suggested as the driving force behind the process of aging as early as the 1950s. Here new insights into cellular metabolism were decisive. Denham Harman hypothesized that free oxygen radicals continually attack the constituent parts of the cell, such as the genome, proteins and fatty acids [16]. He proposed the *free radical theory of aging*, which is popular today due to its comprehensive explanation of the molecular causes of aging. Free radicals are molecules that have an unpaired electron, which makes them highly reactive. So the free radicals modify other molecules, which then often no longer function properly. Although many of the observations of the importance of free radicals in aging are consistent, conclusive proof of the free radical theory has yet remained elusive despite many attempts to date.

Free radicals are not the only way cell structures can be damaged. Cells are constantly exposed to a variety of adverse processes. The causes and consequences of damage, especially damage to the genetic material, will be the subject of a later chapter.

People have always been preoccupied with the problem of aging and death, as shown in our earliest written documents. In the field of biology, the evolutionary biologists were the first to concern themselves with the biology of aging. From evolutionary biology we have learned that the process of aging plays hardly any role in shaping our gene pool. The human body is not designed to last as long as we do these days thanks to medical progress. Thus, the discovery of genes that control aging caused a sensation in aging research. That is what we will be dealing with in the next chapter.

II. Genes Control Aging

II.1. Longevity through genes

Why do molecular biologists like to work with bacteria such as E. coli, or with worms? Thomas Johnson and Cynthia Kenyon showed by implication that there are genes that limit our life span. Aging is thus not just a passive process caused by damage build up.

In the 1960s, biologist Sydney Brenner was looking for a model system that would help explain how nerve cells operate. Model systems are highly important in biological research. You need a species that can be studied in the laboratory. This alone is no easy task, because many biological species are so perfectly adapted to their environment that they cannot thrive in the laboratory. Ideally, results obtained from the study of model organisms can then be applied to other species.

Thus molecular biology began with studies of simple phages and bacteria. The French Nobel laureate Jacques Monod once declared: "Everything that is true in E. coli must also be true in elephants." And indeed, Monod's findings together with François Jacob on the regulation of gene expression in E. coli were of fundamental importance in animals and plants as well. And the more we learned in the last fifty years about the molecular processes of life, the clearer it became that not only the basic building blocks but also the behavior of cells — from unicellular organisms to humans — is very similar, and is thus *evolutionarily conserved.*

Bacteria such as *Escherichia coli* are very easy to grow and to maintain in culture, and so they were the experimental models of choice, particularly in the early years of molecular biology research. In the 1960s there was a trend to move toward eukaryotes such as the yeast *Saccharomyces cerevisiae*, used for thousands of years in baking bread and brewing beer. Later, fungal cells were replaced by human cell cultures, with the isolation of tumor cells being vitally important because cancer cells grow very quickly — even when they are no longer in the body but under suitable growth conditions in cell culture. Studies on all these cells were and still are today extremely significant in building our basic knowledge.

Molecular biology research on whole animals was and still is much more difficult. In order to investigate complex biological functions such as those of the brain, we need to be able to conduct studies on animals. Brenner hit upon the roundworm *Caenorhabditis elegans* [17]. This small nematode worm has proved to be an extraordinarily important model system not only for neurobiology but also for a number of other biological sub-areas. John Sulston recorded what happened to each individual cell as this worm developed from the fertilized egg to adult [18]. Robert Horvitz observed that of all the cells that developed as the worm matured, only 959 survived in the adult animal and 131 cells died by programmed cell death [19]. We will learn more about cell death later on.

In the mid-1980s, biologist Michael Klaas focused on how a nematode worm changed throughout its life. He noticed that certain mutants survived longer than "normal" or wild type worms. We call it a "mutant" when a life form, in this case a nematode, carries a change, that is, a mutation (from the Latin *mutatio*, "change"), in a gene. Klaas called this particular mutant *age-1*, even though it was not initially clear which gene, or perhaps even several genes, were actually changed in the *age-1* mutant animal[1]. Klaas assumed that the *age-1* mutant lived longer because it produced fewer offspring. This conclusion stemmed from the fact that Klaas was only studying worms that could not reproduce. This whole question only became really interesting once T. E. Johnson showed that the inability to reproduce is not a decisive factor in the *age-1* mutants' longer life spans [20]. So instead of a simple redistribution of resources — away from reproduction and toward the preservation of bodily functions — it became clear that there are genes that could limit life spans — and such a gene must have been defective in the *age-1* mutant.

Then Cynthia Kenyon discovered in the 1990s that a further mutant, which was known as *daf-2*, also lived twice as long as a normal roundworm [21]. When normal worms were only feebly lying around after two to three weeks, Kenyon's *daf-2* worms were still quick and lively. Under

---

1 In scientific nomenclature C. elegans genes are named with italicized three (and sometimes four) letters, a dash and a number. The corresponding proteins have the same name but in capital letters and not italicized. For humans usually capital letters are used to symbolize gene (in italics) and protein names.

laboratory conditions, such nematodes generally live for about 20 days, while *daf-2* mutants lived on average 42 days. And they move, are agile and produce nearly as many offspring as completely normal roundworms. So the *daf-2* worms practically enjoyed the secret of eternal youth.

We might well ask, why don't all roundworms share in this genetic fountain of youth? Why in the world should there ever be genes that put a limit on the life span? Wouldn't all worms be better off if they didn't have this destructive gene? To answer the question of why genes place a limit on life, we have to look into evolutionary biology. What happens when a normal *wild type* worm competes with a *daf-2* mutant — who will win? Let's set up a competition between an ordinary worm and a *daf-2* mutant in the laboratory. Both animals produce offspring that reproduce in turn. After a few generations, we find that the population consists almost entirely of *wild type* animals. The *daf-2* mutants lose; they are dying out. The big disadvantage of long-lived animals is that they take more time to produce progeny. While the normal worm needs only a few days to send two to three hundred young into the world, the *daf-2* mutant needs far longer. The next generation of *wild type* animals has reached sexual maturity before most of the descendants of the *daf-2* mutants. As Medawar already noted, when it comes to evolution as a form of competition, it's not how long an individual lives that counts but how successfully it can pass on its genes to future generations.

The *daf-2* mutants should still provide more insights into the biology of aging. At the time when Kenyon made her observations, it was already known that during worms' development changes in the *daf-2* gene could trigger them to enter a so-called "dauer diapause" stage, where their metabolism is relatively inactive; if they remain in this state of arrested development, they live longer but do not reproduce. The wild type can also enter into this phase if they do not find enough food during their growth stage and they receive a "hunger signal" from other worms in their vicinity. It was also discovered that a further mutation, called *daf-16*, could eliminate the formation of permanent "dauer" stages in *daf-2* mutants; it can quash or genetically suppress the *daf-2* mutation. Kenyon was able to demonstrate that the extended life span of the *daf-2* mutants was completely reversed by the further *daf-16* mutation. And this was the decisive observation because it provided the first proof that the extended lifetime was regulated by a genetic mechanism.

Johnson's and Kenyon's discoveries are regarded as revolutionary in our understanding of aging. It was previously assumed that aging was a passive process, which was caused by the accumulation of damage. Now it was recognized that there are genes that can regulate life spans. But that a single gene could have such a serious impact on life expectancy, that a change in a single gene was sufficient to double a life span, was hitherto unthinkable.

The importance of genes in determining life expectancy can be easily illustrated, if we consider that each species has a typical maximum life span. Even though environmental influences can affect the length of a life, as we shall see, the differences in life span between distinct species — which by definition possess distinct gene pools — are far greater.

II.2. The first genetic mechanisms of longevity

Now it's time to get to know the receptors — the eyes and ears of the cell, which open or close the door to the brain's messengers. You'll also get acquainted with the daf-2 gene, which regulates communication between visitors and hosts, and the proteins that, as tools of the cell, determine how long we live.

Subsequently Kenyon in San Francisco and Gary Ruvkun in Boston determined which genes were altered in the *daf-2* and *daf-16* mutants. It turned out that the *daf-2* gene encodes a receptor protein (remember, genes "encode" the information through the formation of proteins) that receives signals on the surface of a cell and forwards them into the cell.

Receptors are the eyes and ears of a cell. A receptor is a protein that usually sticks out from the cell membrane to receive signals from the environment. Cells have a myriad of different receptors, which in turn can recognize each specific messenger substance. The messengers give signals from cell to cell, or they can also transfer signals to the whole animal. In people, for example, growth hormone is formed in the brain and then travels through the bloodstream to the remotest tissues to convey their message — to get the cells to grow.

The receptor protein DAF-2 binds messengers that are similar to human insulin. The roundworm has dozens of different insulin-like messengers, but only a few so far known to bind to the DAF-2 receptor. When a messenger molecule binds to a receptor, normally the receptor is activated, but it may also be deactivated. An activated receptor then sends the signal further into the cell. This often happens through highly complex downstream signaling pathways within the cell. These can form whole signaling networks and interact with other signaling pathways. The signals can in turn activate or inactivate proteins downstream.

If a mutation reduces the activity of the DAF-2 receptor, the worm lives longer; but only so long as the DAF-16 protein is present, because a mutation in the *daf-16* gene suppresses the longevity effect of the *daf-2* mutants. So, now we just need to find out what miracles the DAF-16 protein is working that could end up doubling the life span of the animal. In roundworms, a *daf-2* mutation and the DAF-16 protein do something so fundamentally important that the worm can survive longer. And humans, by the way, have genes that are surprisingly similar to worms' *daf-2* and *daf-16*.

Around the turn of the millennium, Johnson employed a very important method that allows proteins in a living cell to be observed: the green fluorescent protein, GFP for short. GFP is a protein that was obtained from a jellyfish in the 1960s; after being stimulated by blue to ultraviolet light, it turns green. Martin Chalfie, Osamu Shimomura and Roger Tsien discovered that the GFP gene could be attached to a gene from another organism, a trick that won them the 2008 Nobel Prize in Chemistry. With the fusion of GFP, any protein could now be visualized in a live cell, a tissue or in a whole organism. Johnson generated nematodes in which the GFP gene had been appended to the *daf-16* gene. Now Johnson could track where the DAF-16::GFP fusion protein was in each cell in the living roundworm at any time. In the normal worm, at first, this was rather less than spectacular: DAF-16::GFP was outside of the nucleus, somewhere in the cytoplasm. But it was a very different matter in the long-lived *daf-2* mutants: Suddenly the cell nuclei glowed before him, bright with GFP-labeled DAF-16. Johnson also could observe nuclear DAF-16::GFP in normal wild type worms as soon as he put them in stressful situations; for worms, stress can be anything from a higher temperature to the presence of toxic substances or lack of food. And under each of those conditions, the DAF-16 protein accumulated in the cell nucleus. So DAF-16 performs a function in the cell nucleus, and this function is necessary for the *daf-2* mutant's extraordinarily prolonged life. What does the DAF-16 do in the cell nucleus?

Interestingly, the DAF-16 protein is a so-called a *transcription factor*. What makes a transcription factor? As we learned earlier, transcription is the process by which the hereditary information, DNA, is transmitted into mRNA molecules. This transmission is necessary for translating the genetic information that is safely stored in the nucleus into proteins like enzymes that are synthesized in the cytoplasm. Whether a gene is read (i.e., switched on) or repressed (that is, switched off) is determined by transcription factors. Transcription factors are the decisive proteins that determine which scores from the symphonies of the genome are played. If DAF-16 is in the cell nucleus, the orchestra of genes plays a long Adagio; and the animal ages in slow motion.

Since every cell contains all the genetic material, it is absolutely necessary to establish precisely which genes are active and which are inactive. Otherwise there would be complete chaos in the cellular processes. That is precisely why the many different transcription factors are so important. They determine which genes are on and which are off at any time, and even more, they specify how much mRNA a gene produces, and when.

This ensures that cells in the scalp produce keratin or muscle cells produce the structural parts of the muscle fibers. The combination of transcription factors thus determines the function of a cell.

With the realization that the activation of DAF-16 extends the life span, scientists suddenly realized that the DAF-16-controlled genes influence the process of aging. By now, hundreds of genes were found to be regulated by DAF-16; and even more transcription factors have been found that can alter the life span together with DAF-16 or independently. We will discuss in the following section the very processes that enable an organism to live especially long. But before that, we'll focus on the question of what significance these long-lived roundworms may hold for other living beings, especially for us humans. This question has, of course, been closely studied ever since Kenyon's discovery.

II.3. Genetic defects, growth hormones and their importance for aging — in mice and humans

The Laron Syndrome is named after the Israeli pediatric endocrinologist Zvi Laron, who conducted research in the late 1950s on people who were normal size when their life began but then grew very slowly due to a genetic defect that interferes with the growth process. In a mountain village in Ecuador, there live dozens of dwarves. A researcher wondered: Could these little people be carrying the key to a long life?

To prolong the life of a worm is, scientifically, certainly interesting. But the real question is whether these processes also are relevant for us human beings. To address this question, first we'll study the equivalent genes in another no less important *model system*, fruit flies. The fruit fly *Drosophila melanogaster* was used as early as the 1920s by the great geneticist Herman Muller to track hereditary characteristics. Muller studied how white and red eyes, and mutilated and normal wings, have been inherited. Through these experiments, he came to the realization that genes are inherited through chromosomes, one of the fundamental insights of genetics.

D. melanogaster has become one of the most important tools of the geneticist and is today a central model system of modern biology. An equivalent of the *daf-2*-mutant worm was established with flies carrying the *chico* mutation. The *chico* gene encodes a protein that receives and forwards signals from the insulin receptor, i.e., the fly version of *daf-2*. Similar to *daf-2*-worms, flies with a mutation in the *chico* gene live longer [22].

The next step in exploring whether the longevity of nematodes has any relevance for other animals had thus been made, because it was now clear that the genetic mechanism that determines life span is *evolutionarily conserved*, in other words, it is retained throughout evolutionary history.

To see whether observations in nematode worms and fruit flies also have relevance for higher animals, experiments are usually carried out in mice. The house mouse, *mus musculus*, is one of the most widely used animal models in the study of disease processes. For many decades mice have been bred under controlled conditions in laboratories worldwide. The mice are mated within a strain, so that there are many strains of mice that are totally inbred and stable. This is important and desirable in order to ensure that research on disease genes, for example, can be carried out against the same genetic background, irrespective of whether the mouse to be studied is kept in Germany, Japan or the United States of America. Of course, people have been breeding mice in the same way as humans have been breeding their farm animals for ten thousand years, almost inadvertently selecting for those who breed early and have many progeny. This is due to the fact that the animals are bred young and the offspring come mostly from young parents. In the protected environment of the laboratory, mice can live from twenty-four to about thirty-six months. In the wild, few mice survive longer than eight months since the winter cold is a big problem for them. Interestingly, though, wild mice that are captured, free of inbreeding and selection for early birth, survive even longer in the protected laboratory than the strains of laboratory mice. However, studies using wild mice are often very difficult to interpret, because their life histories as well as genetic composition are difficult to reconstruct. Studies on wild mice are in fact rare. Richard Miller, a biologist working in Michigan, is an enthusiastic advocate of animal studies in their natural environment, especially mice in the wild. Life history of the animals under natural conditions can be tediously followed by catch-and-recapture experiments. Nonetheless, there are many limitations for studying wild animals, for example when one wishes to understand the role that particular genes have in diseases, because such an analysis inevitably requires comparisons within a defined genetic background in order to single out the role of any specific gene.

The first long-lived mice had already been bred in laboratories in the 1920s. Here's what happened: George Snell isolated some dwarf mice after birth, and at first they looked quite normal. But after two weeks their bodies stopped growing entirely [23]. They only reached about a quarter of the body weight of normal mice. Later, in the 1950s, the Ames dwarf mice were isolated in the Ames laboratories of the University of Iowa. At first there was not much interest in understanding the entire life cycle of the dwarf mice. It was even assumed that these mice were inherently short-lived. It turns out that this was due to the fact that the breeding conditions were not up to today's standards. By giving them better treatment, Holly Brown-Borg and Andrzej Bartke were able to conduct a more detailed investigation of the life span of the dwarf mice [24]. They lived a whole year longer than the normal species, and two of the female dwarf mice even set a new record for mouse longevity, reaching the age of four years.

The Snell and Ames dwarf mice are small because they are missing different genes, which are necessary for the development of the pituitary gland. The pituitary gland serves the brain as an endocrine organ; by releasing hormones it regulates various processes throughout the entire body, including growth, reproduction, and metabolism. Reduced body growth is the most obvious: if insufficient growth hormone is produced due to a poorly formed pituitary— the mice remain small.

Next, John Kopchick demonstrated that growth hormone is a decisive factor for both reduced growth and extended life. Kopchick developed a mouse that carried a mutation in the growth hormone receptor itself. This mouse had completely normal levels of pituitary hormones. The mere absence of the receptor that detects the growth hormone was sufficient for the mice to remain just as small as the Snell and Ames dwarf mice and, what is even more interesting for us, of course, they enjoyed a long life.

Which function of the growth hormone is essential for extending life? The growth hormone receptor that Kopchick examined regulates yet another important messenger substance: The production of what is called "Insulin-like growth factor-1" or IGF-1 for short. In fact, mice with decreased IGF-1 receptor activity also live longer [25]. And now comes the best part: The IGF-1 receptor is the direct equivalent of the *daf-2* gene in Kenyon's nematodes. The decreased activity of insulin-like signaling helps prolong life in species from simple nematode roundworms all the way up to mammals.

The question immediately arises: Is this also the case in humans?

Jaime Guevara-Aguirre, an endocrinologist who was working on metabolic and hormonal disorders, visited a village in the mountains of Ecuador in 1987 where a striking number of diminutive people live. The men were about 4'7" feet tall and the women only 4'3" feet. It turned out that a mutation in the growth hormone receptor was a contributing factor, just as it was in the mice that John Kopchick had studied. And just like the dwarf mice, these people in Ecuador also showed greatly reduced body growth. How does that relate to their life expectancy?

Together with a researcher on aging, Valter Longo from the University of Southern California, Guevara-Aguirre (who was originally from southern Ecuador himself) studied their backgrounds[26]. These folks were probably descendants of Sephardic Jews who had fled to Ecuador from persecution by the Inquisition in Spain, and in the seclusion of this village the defective gene was passed on from generation to generation. The researchers had to refer to the medical records. Of course, the life expectancy of Ecuadorian villagers is not the same as that of the average North American from Longo's environment. But not all the inhabitants of this mountain village were dwarves. Some of their partners and siblings shared a partial mutation in the growth hormone, while others had normal growth hormone receptors and grew to a normal body size. Thus, the two researchers had enough small and normal-sized people to study aging and disease among people with and without the growth hormone receptor.

To the disappointment of the researcher on aging, the short-statured Ecuadorians experienced no increase in life expectancy. Nevertheless, their biographies showed astonishing differences. The causes of death differed dramatically from those of the normal-growth villagers. The smaller people were far more likely to suffer accidents. Many of them had alcohol problems. Also they tended to develop epilepsy. On the other hand, they were immune to cancer and also rarely developed diabetes. Apparently, the absence of growth hormone receptors was an effective protection against two important diseases associated with aging.

In our latitudes, too, people who lack this receptor also appear again and again with severe growth defects, although never in such high numbers as in the aforementioned village in South America. These people suffer from Laron Syndrome, first described in the 1950s by an Israeli pediatric endocrinologist, Zvi Laron. The example of these individuals with Laron Syndrome gives us a hint that the results from studies on mice and other animal models can bring us important insights into the origins of various diseases and disorders.

Human aging, however, is subject to a great many influences, which are quite different from those affecting animals kept in the laboratory, for example. A reduction of growth signals can evidently counteract cancer development in mice as well as in humans. Cancer is a disease that is particularly difficult to treat, and the risk of developing cancer increases dramatically with age: age itself is a major risk factor for cancer. As we grow older, our bodies produce less growth hormone and IGF-1, and this reduction is apparently one of our body's natural mechanisms to counteract the increasing risk of cancer. Preventive therapies could start with circulating growth factors in the bloodstream. It has not yet been proven whether altering the balance of growth factors will also help extend life.

We do know something about using hormone supplements as a medical treatment, for instance hormone replacement therapy for women in menopause. A hormone deficit can have serious health consequences. In addition to low estrogen levels, a low level of growth hormone also contributes to the development of osteoporosis, because both these hormones are important for bone stability. Hormone treatments can also carry risks, notably an increased risk of cancer. Any time hormone therapy is contemplated, it is essential to accurately weigh the pros and cons in each individual case. The complexity of the interaction of hormones in the human body should not be underestimated. For a complete understanding of these interactions, we will have to conduct many studies, especially in mouse models.

It is no longer impossible to foresee effective interventions to prevent age-related diseases such as cancer and diabetes, and even to prolong a healthy life. Animal studies have already proven that it is fundamentally feasible. Disease prevention among humans is indeed a priority goal in the field of Biomedical Aging Research. Manipulating the hormone balance offers great opportunities, but the consequences need to be well understood in order to ensure that overall the effect on human health is positive.

To identify genetic variations that may endow certain people with a special longevity, gerontologists and geriatricians, biologists and medical researchers dealing with the question of aging around the world have been seeking out people whose families have included surprising numbers of centenarians. Centenarian studies are underway in Germany, Japan, England, the Netherlands, the USA and many other countries. In the groups of centenarians that are being studied, longevity is passed from generation to generation. Every conceivable parameter is being investigated: growth factors are measured in the blood system; the expression of genes is assessed; genetic material is being sequenced[1]; health status is analyzed. At the same time, the centenarians are often compared with their life partners who share the same living conditions, diet and habits. Whatever it is that differs between the centenarians and their partners, so the logic goes, may be the key to longevity.

Longevity research on centenarians has already been fruitful. Variations have been found in genes that had already come to light during longevity trials with simple animal models. In Japanese as well as in German centenarian populations, people who live longer showed changes in the *FOXO* gene. This *FOXO* gene is the human equivalent of precisely that *daf-16* transcription factor we know from the nematode [27], [28]. And a variation in the gene for the IGF-1 receptor, the equivalent of the *daf-2* gene in the nematode, was found in a US study of long-lived Ashkenazi Jews [29].

These results suggest that the same genes that control longevity in simple animals also affect the human life span, and thus they could form the basis of *anti-aging* medicine. Yet, finding these genetic variations in centenarians still does not prove that these genes are responsible for their

---

1 By sequencing the genome, the exact sequence of ATGC in the genome is determined. For example, particularly long-lived people carry certain variants of genes responsible for their longevity.

long life expectancy. Moreover, this long life is showing up generation after generation, arguing against the simple explanation based on individual genetic variations, because one would expect the genes that are inherited from the parent who did not have an unusually long life to offset the effect of the long-life genes. It is therefore possible that even non-genetic factors, so-called epigenetics (from Greek *epi* "beyond"),[1] are at the root of these centenarians' long lives. It is also possible that significant events in the centenarians' lives have been overlooked when comparing them with their partners. The study of human longevity is sure to bring to light interesting new information regarding how average people can age in a healthier way.

---

1 Epigenetics refers to controls of the function of genes that do not reside in the DNA ATGC code. These can be, for example, chemical modifications to the DNA itself, which regulate the expression of genes.

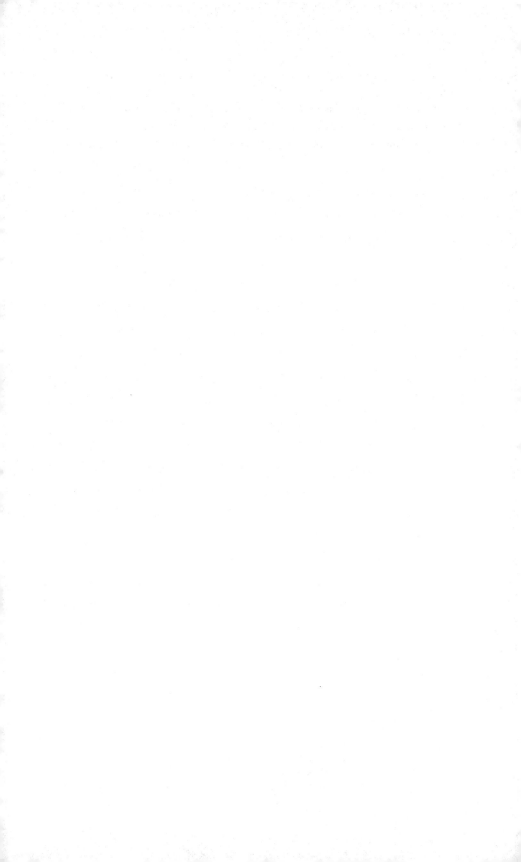

III. The Process of Human Aging

The race to decode the human genome culminated in 2001 with the publication of the genome sequence — a kind of blueprint of the human being, if you will.

But our genome is attacked by many factors and is constantly changing. Some modifications lead to diseases. To counteract this challenge, repair mechanisms have also emerged in evolution.

How can we test the role of genes in human aging? We'll be looking for answers to these questions in this third chapter. As we have seen, we can analyze the functions of genes by producing mutants in animal models, and even in mammals. We have already looked at mutations in nematodes, flies and mice that carry a modified sequence of a gene, i.e., a genetic change, which is called a mutation. Learning how to produce mutations was a crucial step forward for biological research in the 20th century. In mice we can now disable any gene and thus produce animals with a defective gene. If a certain phenotype or trait occurs, such as a growth defect, or if the mouse mutant develops a disease, one can infer that the mutated gene is important for growth or for preventing a specific disease.

Mutations in humans are the cause of hereditary diseases. Some rare genetic diseases that lead to premature aging of the patient give us information about the genetic causes of human aging. What are these mutations, what do these genes do?

Mutations can arise spontaneously and be passed on for generations. There would be no evolution if no mutations had taken place after the first DNA molecule was formed. Mutations enabled the first form of life to evolve into the whole spectrum of species diversity over billions of years. And every person carries mutations in his or her genome (the term genome refers to the totality of the genes of an organism). Although one person's genome is very similar to another person's, only the genomes of identical twins are completely identical — and even there, strictly speaking, only just when they are created in the womb. No two people have the exact same genome. Everyone has variations, be they ever so small. That is why humans, just like most animal species, are so different from one another.

Most variations in the genome sequence, i.e., the ATGC sequence in the DNA, have no consequences. Only a very small part of our genome contains genes — surprising as that sounds at first. The human genome comprises the total stock of base pairs in the DNA of an individual; it consists of 3 billion DNA building blocks, the *nucleotides* with their *bases* A, T, G and C linked via ribose molecules to long strands of *chromosomes*. The length of nucleotides a gene can contain varies greatly, from a few hundred to thousands of different sequences of A, T, G and C.

Only in the last few years did it become possible to sequence a complete genome, especially one as big as the human genome, that is, to determine in what order the nucleotides are arranged in the DNA. With the Human Genome Project of the 1990s, scientists had set themselves the target of establishing the sequence of nucleotides across the entire human genome. First they tried it with smaller genomes, from simpler organisms like bacteria. The first animal to have its genome sequenced was none other than our little friend, the nematode. The *C. elegans* genome was the successful test-run for the Human Genome Project.

The multi-billion dollar publicly funded Human Genome Project soon ran into commercial competition from Craig Venter, a biochemist turned entrepreneur, and his Celera Corporation; for him, no goal seemed too high to shoot for. Although initially this private competition was met with a certain level of resentment, perhaps even contempt, it turned out to be a blessing. Now the race was on to complete the human genome sequence. If Celera had won, there was the prospect that a corporation would seek to obtain the patent on all human genes — a scenario straight out of a horror movie. This drove the public project to gear up and get the job done. The substantial funding that flowed into the two projects led to rapid technical advances in the sequencing machines. And by the year 2001, they did it. Celera and the Human Genome Project published the sequence of the human genome [30], [31], a milestone in the history of "knowledgeable" man, *Homo sapiens*, because now we know the code — the blueprint — of man.

In the following years the sequence definition has been further refined, with the focus shifting more and more to the correct interpretation of the sequence. In the end, determining the sequence was only a necessary first step in getting to understand the human genome. For the sequence to make sense, to interpret it, is a challenge for the genome researchers even today.

Perhaps the most surprising finding was the relatively small number of genes in the human genome. In the 1990s it was still assumed that our genome might encode up to 100,000 genes, while today's understanding is that there are only about 20,000 to 25,000 human genes [32]. This figure is especially startling when we recall that even the simple nematode, with just 959 cells, has about 20,000 genes.[1]

Even after the human genome was "decoded," progress was made not only in interpreting the genome, but also in the speed at which the sequencing machines were improved. Sequencing that just a few years ago could take months can now be done within a day. The Human Genome Project started with the genomes of just a few people. At the current rate of technological development, we will soon be able to sequence the genome of every human being. That will enable us to find important clues to whatever diseases concern us personally.[2]

Determining the human genome sequence is enormously important as we search for the causes of genetic diseases. Mutations arise due to damage to the genetic material. DNA is not completely stable; it can be chemically modified. Every day of our life, DNA damage is produced in each of our cells tens of thousands of times. Our genome is attacked by many different factors. The skin is exposed to the sun's ultraviolet radiation, which reacts directly with the nucleotides of the DNA and can alter its structure. This is why sun bathing leads to skin cancer — but more about that later. Even the natural metabolism in our cells can cause DNA damage, for example by releasing reactive oxygen, a radical, as mentioned earlier. DNA is subject to many chemical attacks and even to cosmic radiation — we are exposed to it constantly, and especially at higher altitudes when flying — so that ongoing DNA damage is inevitable.

Since genome damage has been a part of life throughout evolution, DNA repair systems evolved already in the earliest organisms. These repair systems are extremely important to ensure that most DNA damage can be corrected, and, indeed, the bulk of DNA damage can be repaired quite well. But nothing is perfect, and DNA repair systems can make a mistake. An error

---

1 The significant difference between the genes in the human genome compared to the nematode genome lies in the very diverse variants in which genes are expressed. This allows the limited number of human genes to encode a large variety of proteins — that accounts for the estimated 100,000 different proteins that are formed.

2 Knowing your own "personal" genome is no longer limited by the actual sequencing. It is far more difficult to derive a correct prediction of the risk of disease from the many variations in genes that every person carries.

in the repair can mean that the DNA sequence is not accurately restored to the way it was before the damage. And right there, we see a mutation.

Mutations can occur in any cell. If a mutation occurs in a single-cell organism, such as a baker's yeast cell, all the descendants of this cell will exhibit the mutation. In the human body, mutations can have many different consequences. Nerve cells are all formed during our development and they never divide again. If a nerve cell dies, it cannot be replaced. Any mutation arising in a nerve cell vanishes with it. Cells in the intestine and skin, on the other hand, are constantly replaced. The intestine and skin have very active stem cells, and they constantly produce new intestinal and skin cells. If a mutation occurs for example in a skin stem cell, all the skin cells emerging from it carry the mutation. But if a mutation occurs in a *differentiated* cell, for example a specialized skin cell, it usually doesn't make a difference because the skin cell will soon be shed and will be replaced by a newly produced cell anyway.

All mutations that occur within the somatic cells have no impact beyond our own bodies. They disappear, either when the mutated cell dies or at the latest with the death of the body. It is quite a different matter with mutations in the germ line: the germ cells do pass on their genetic information to future cells.

Germ cells are therefore particularly sensitive to DNA damage. Sperm often die, if they detect DNA damage in their genome. The ova, or eggs, on the other hand, are particularly good at repairing their genome. Nevertheless, mutations that are inherited can occur. Such mutations remain in the human gene pool for a very long time.

Normally, hereditary mutations have only little consequence because two copies of each chromosome and thus the whole genome are present in each of our cells. We inherit one set of chromosomes from our mother, the second from our father. The only famous exception is the chromosome that determines our gender; men have one X and one Y chromosome, while women have two Xs. If a mutation is inherited from one parent, we usually get the normal gene from the other parent.

Most mutations do not show up as long as a normal copy of the gene is present. Such mutations are called *recessive*. However, there are also *dominant* mutations that take over even if a normal copy of the equivalent gene is also present. Most mutations are harmless. They concern, for example, the color of eyes and hair. There may be dominant gene variants such as, for example, brown eye color, and recessive gene variants such as blue eye color.

Mutations can also cause serious hereditary diseases. Such mutations are recessive because if they were dominant, they would quickly disappear from the gene pool. Anyone carrying a dominant mutation that causes severe illness will become ill and die. A recessive mutation, on the other hand, can lie dormant in our genome and be passed on from generation to generation. If both parents have such a recessive mutation, the normal variant of the gene may be omitted from the child, so that both the maternal and paternal chromosomes contain the mutated gene.

Such genetic diseases are more common in regions where people marry among close relatives. In such cases, there is less variety in the gene pool of the population. Thus there are many sources of the same gene variants and thus the same recessive mutations. Often this results in whole families being affected by hereditary diseases. With the modern methods of genome sequencing that have been developed in the last few years, it is becoming possible to identify more and more of the mutations that cause rare hereditary diseases.

Identifying the genetic mutations that cause human hereditary diseases is not only critically important for the understanding of diseases, but it also sheds light on the normal functioning of the human body. If a person suffers from an inherited disease, one can now look in the genome to see which gene has a mutation. By this means, one may be able to tell which variations of genes are common to people who either age too fast or who have particularly long lives. This is exactly the goal of the field of human genetics.

The identification of disease genes is already making good progress when it comes to so-called *monogenic* diseases. "Monogenic" refers to hereditary diseases that are caused by a defect in one single gene (*mono* = "one"). The sequence of this gene is different in the patient than it is in his siblings who do not have the hereditary disease. Imagine, then, that certain genes are necessary to keep the body functioning until old age; one would expect the defects in these genes to accelerate the aging process. This is, in fact, the case in premature aging syndromes, called *progerias*.

Investigating hereditary diseases that influence aging has led to considerable breakthroughs in understanding the process of aging itself, as well as the diseases and infirmities that typically come with aging. In the following section, we'll look more closely at these hereditary diseases of premature aging.

III.1. Premature aging: When children are already aged

In this chapter we meet a few 'old boys': The Hutchinson-Gilford Progeria Syndrome and its younger siblings the Werner Syndrome, Blooms Syndrome and Rothmund-Thomson Syndrome. They explain what happens when the "helicase" fails to repair a car traveling at full speed, and why a diseased trunkful of hereditary material gives you wrinkles and gray hair.

Jonathan Hutchinson was a Jack-of-all-trades in the British medical establishment of the late 19th century. There are not many diseases that he missed thoroughly investigating. He was an eye doctor and a general practitioner, and he had many ideas about sexually transmitted diseases, and for fighting syphilis, which was a widespread scourge at the time — he recommended preventive circumcision. A man of his times, he also suggested that where excessive masturbation was a problem, castration seemed like a viable solution. But the London doctor made a discovery that landed him in the annals of scientific history: In 1886 Jonathan Hutchinson conducted ground-breaking research on a patient who suffered a severe case of premature aging.

This premature aging syndrome was named after Hutchinson and the surgeon Hastings Gilford who came out with his own independent analysis of the same disease just a short while later. The Hutchinson-Gilford Progeria Syndrome (HGPS) becomes evident in early childhood. (The name "Progeria" comes from pro "before, sooner" + geron "an elder," "an old man" — as in geriatrics, healthcare for elderly people.) Children who have HGPS exhibit pronounced growth disorders, deformities, skin that is pitted, hardened or scarred (fibrosis) — and hair loss. HGPS patients usually die by the age of 13 due to cardiovascular disorders. The cause of this dreadful disease was brought to light about one hundred years later, in 2003, as a result of genetic research on HGPS.

Francis Collins is a researcher, chemist, geneticist, doctor and currently serves as Director of the (US) National Institutes of Health (NIH), which in addition to its own huge institutes near Washington, DC, is also the largest funding organization for American medical research. Collins looks like a geek, but there are many sides to his personality. In his free time he plays hard rock, with folks like Joe Perry of Aerosmith, and he likes to ride his motorcycle — he prefers big, loud engines. An evangelical Christian originally from Virginia, he was met with a lot of skepticism from his American colleagues when President Obama made him the most powerful scientist in the NIH leadership. Nevertheless, Collins clearly positioned himself to move forward in researching embryonic stem cells, which many ultra-religious Americans see as a sin.

In the 1970s Collins was a young doctor at Yale University in Connecticut, where he came across Meg, a young woman 23 years of age. Light as a feather, and bald, Meg suffered from premature aging. Collins could not accept the fact that he was unable to help this patient and relieve her suffering; she died from HGPS in 1985. The hidden cause of this disease preyed on his mind. With the modern techniques of genome analysis available since the 1990s, it has become more and more feasible to identify precisely which genome sections lie behind various hereditary diseases, and studying twenty victims of this extremely rare syndrome, Collins and his team noticed a difference in their *lamin-A* gene. This mutation leads to a faulty reading of the gene itself. Lamin-A is part of the nucleus of a cell structure, and the HGPS mutation damages its stability. The nucleus has to be able to withstand certain mechanical stresses; muscle cells, for instance, have to be able to tolerate the strain put on a muscle. And when the cell cannot bear up under this pressure, its essential biological processes are disturbed.

Interestingly, these abnormal forms of *lamin-A* gene are found increasingly often in cells of normal people as they age. This suggests that the reduced stability of the nucleus that causes the premature aging of HGPS patients could also play a causal role in the normal aging process.

Since the genetic cause of HGPS was found, researchers have been able to get a better insight into the molecular relationships between the stability of the cell nucleus and the aging process. The cells of HGPS patients respond to mechanical loads like an extremely sensitive tissue that is subjected to pressure. This was not really apparent at first, because cells held in laboratory conditions normally are not exposed to mechanical loads the way some tissues in the body are during physical activity.

The cell nucleus has long been understood to be the central protected area where the genetic material is stored in each cell. All processes involving the genes are done in the nucleus. The cell nucleus is where DNA replication takes place (the duplication of DNA before cell division) and transcription (reading the DNA in order for it to be rewritten in mRNA during gene expression). If the nucleus is not entirely stable, this has a direct impact on the stability of the genome itself.[1]

In HGPS, the genome itself is unstable. For example, there are more breaks in the strands of DNA. These DNA breaks activate a highly complex damage response mechanism. Such damage response mechanisms are immensely important for aging, and we will deal with this in more detail later on. But first of all, let's look closer at the premature-aging syndromes.

In his dissertation in the early 20th century, Otto Werner, a medical student in Kiel, Germany, described four brothers and sisters who, although they were not even thirty years of age, already looked quite elderly. The Werner syndrome is probably the best-known premature aging syndrome. Premature aging syndromes are also called Segmental Progeria. Here,

---

1 It is thought that a part of the DNA repair and transcription takes place directly underneath the envelope of the cell nucleus. The envelope of the cell nucleus not only protects, but it has pores through which the RNA and proteins from the cell nucleus are transported to the cell plasma. Conversely, all proteins used in the cell nucleus must pass inward through the nuclear pores. The cell nucleus is thus not only the vault that holds the genome but also the logistics center of the cell.

segmental means that it's not the entire organism that shows signs of aging, but only certain segments, specific tissues and organs, show accelerated aging. This is an important issue as we seek to understand the causes of aging. The segmental appearance of aging means that different biological processes affect the maintenance of cell function in different tissues.

The biochemist Larry Loeb has shown that in Werner Syndrome patients, the mutated gene is a DNA-helicase. Helicases are thus named because they are proteins that open and unwind the DNA double helix. Helicases are critically important, because the two strands of DNA have to be separated from each other each time the genome is duplicated. The DNA has to be replicated, that is, copied, with every cell division. In addition, DNA also has to be opened during certain repairs. The Werner helicase plays an important role in this process. If it doesn't work, some forms of damage to the genome cannot be repaired properly.

Abnormalities in helicases (like Werner's helicase) have also been recognized as causative in other segmental progeroid syndromes. The Bloom helicase causes the syndrome of that name (described by New York dermatologist David Bloom for the first time in the 1950s in patients with severe growth disorders and skin dysplasia). The Rothmund-Thomson Syndrome (RTS) is also attributed to a malfunctioning helicase. RTS patients first experience growth disturbance and they form a rash on their skin when exposed to sunlight. As this progeria develops, patients are subject to very typical aging phenomena such as cataracts — which is like a gray star clouding the lens of the eye — and soon their hair turns gray, too. These patients also typically suffer from early cancer.

Knowing the molecular causes of Werner, Blooms and Rothmund-Thomson Syndromes has made it clear that preserving genetic material is a key element in achieving a long life. In recent years, more and more of the rarely occurring progeria have been investigated. In many cases, the underlying genetic defect has already been recognized; the very genes that when defective cause premature aging have repeatedly been found to play an important role in repairing the genome.

Genome repair is a highly complex process. There are many hundreds of different ways the DNA can be damaged; and, the biggest challenge for the repair mechanisms is to detect damage when it occurs. If you can imagine which dynamic processes of the genome are involved, you might have some sense of how difficult it is to identify damage in the form of small chemical changes in the nucleotides. There are many hundreds of different types of damage. When the DNA is copied (replicated), or transcribed into RNA, it must be opened by helicases. This process leads to changes in the DNA's three-dimensional helix structure. These normal changes in the

DNA structure must be distinguished from changes caused by damage.[1] Our DNA is approximately 6 feet long; in other words, the DNA of each cell is a hundred thousand times longer than the diameter of a typical cell. Therefore, the DNA must be tightly packed in the cell nucleus. The DNA is present in the cell in various deformations that can change dynamically, for example when a gene is activated or when the DNA needs to be replicated. In this dynamic context, DNA damage has to be detected and repaired, which is a little like repairing a car while speeding along the highway.

III.2. How cells react to DNA damage: checkpoints and cancer

In this chapter, we see what happens when DNA gets broken; it creates problems for the mother cells with their dissimilar daughters.

"Checkpoints" struggle with growth hormones to control the degenerate new cells. They receive support from the p53 gene. They neutralize dangerous cells by inhibiting their action, de-activating them, or discarding them; this makes them harmless, while the Bcl2 gene saves suicidal cells — but not human lives.

The type of DNA damage most commonly seen is when there are small breaks in one of the two strands of the DNA's double helix. Such fractures occur by the tens of thousands in each of our body's cells every day. If only one strand is broken, it can be linked together again by specialized proteins called DNA ligases (from the Latin *ligare*, "connect").

Double strand breaks are far more serious, because the ends of the fractures can move away from each other. If two double-strand breaks occur on the same chromosome, there is a risk that the whole genome section will be lost. If two different chromosomes are broken at the same time, a faulty chromosome fusion can occur: the wrong ends are joined together. DNA double strand breaks are extremely dangerous for the cell. This is especially true when a cell divides while one of its chromosomes is broken. The chromosome sets may be distributed unequally to the resulting cells, a phenomenon called aneuploidy. We'll see just how dangerous such an unequal distribution of chromosomes can be in a later section. The cell has a variety of repair machines for mending double strand breaks, adapted to particular situations. But these repair mechanisms need time in order to do the job properly. The damaged DNA must not be copied and the cell should not divide until the double strand breaks are resolved.

---

1 Because only a small part of our genome encodes genes and each cell reads only certain genes, there are active and inactive parts of the genome. An intestinal cell, for example, does not use the gene for eye color and so such a gene must be switched off in intestinal cells. Because each cell has an entire genome, it is very important to regulate precisely which genes are active and to what extent. The structures of active and inactive parts of the genome are very different.

In the 1980s, baker's yeast was found to show a very specific behavior: after the cells were exposed to DNA damage, they stopped dividing for a while. This behavior has been called cell cycle arrest, i.e., a pause in the division behavior of the yeast cell. Cell division is called the cell cycle because the sequence of processes that make up cell division keeps repeating in an ongoing cycle. Before the cell divides, the genome of the cell is copied so that each daughter cell will receive a full set of chromosomes. After the DNA is copied, or *replicated*, the cell pauses briefly to distribute the chromosomes evenly; then the cell nucleus and finally the entire cell will be divided. After the two daughter cells have separated, the DNA can start duplicating itself again.

The yeast geneticists Leland Hartwell and Ted Weinert introduced the concept of checkpoints. This term describes the behavior of the baker's yeast where the process of cell division goes forward only when the previous cycle has been completed [35]. Thus the cells do not begin to divide until all the chromosomes have been replicated, so that both daughter cells can get the complete set of chromosomes.

Hartwell and Weinert noticed that the cells do not begin to replicate the DNA if they have been treated with ionizing radiation that leads to DNA damage. (We will soon be taking a close look at why ionizing radiation is so dangerous to the DNA.) In cases where the cells had already duplicated the chromosomes and got damaged afterwards, they would not set into motion the process of cell division. At every step on the way, from inactivity to replication of the DNA, from replication of the DNA to the division of the whole cell, there is always a checkpoint that has to be passed at which the cell verifies that the previous step has been completed and that no damage to the chromosomes is present.

Hartwell, Weinert and later an ever-increasing number of other researchers, have been able to use the excellent properties of baker's yeast, *Saccharomyces cerevisiae*, as well as its distant relative the fission yeast, *Schizosaccharomyces pombe*, to clarify how checkpoints work. Fission yeast provided many of the clues to our understanding of the cell cycle, that is, the sequence of the different phases of cell division. [1]

Soon, mutated yeast cells were found, which — in contrast to normal yeast cells– failed to interrupt their cell cycle after they experienced DNA damage. These so-called checkpoint mutants then led researchers to the genes that control the various checkpoints. These checkpoint genes control, for example, whether the replication of the DNA can begin or whether the cell can go ahead and divide, or whether the chromosomes are evenly distributed

---

1 The rod-shaped fission yeast got that name because during cell division it grows at both ends and then splits exactly in the middle. In contrast to this, in baker's yeast the daughter cell forms as a bud on the parent cell and drops off.

to the daughter cells. Since the first checkpoint genes were uncovered in the late 1980s, whole networks of checkpoint genes have been identified.

If the checkpoints do not function properly, the cell does not have enough time to repair its damaged DNA. Therefore, cells whose checkpoints do not work are particularly sensitive to DNA damage. Cells without functioning checkpoints show instability of their genome. And an unstable genome is a very typical feature of cancer cells.

Cancer is a particularly treacherous disease because cancer cells are actually cells of our own body that grow uncontrollably. Cell division itself is obviously an essential process to generate and maintain an organism. Indeed, all our body cells originally came from a single cell, the fertilized egg. In the body of an adult human, stem cells are also continuously undergoing division. Our blood, skin, and intestinal cells must be constantly renewed to keep our body alive.

However, the number of cell divisions must be strictly controlled. This is done by growth hormones that impel the cells to divide, while the checkpoint genes put on the brakes, and together they ensure that each cell splits as often as necessary. The activity of growth hormones and checkpoint genes is precisely regulated in our bodies. Cancerous cells arise when the division of the cells is accelerated by the growth hormones and the cells' checkpoints no longer function. Then the cancer cells divide continually, resulting in the formation of tumors.

If you look at the karyotype of a cancer cell, that is, the number and structure of its chromosomes, you will quickly see that they rarely have a normal set of chromosomes. Non-functioning checkpoints are indeed one of the causes for the development of cancer. Many genes in cancer cells show a host of mutations because malfunctioning checkpoints hamper with the repair of DNA damage. A cancer cell can therefore go on living with DNA damage and can continue to replicate and divide, thus growing into an ever-larger tumor. A cancer cell doesn't need many of the genes anyway, as it doesn't have to form hair or bones or perform any other specialized tasks.

The most frequently mutated gene in cancer cells goes by the innocent-sounding name "p53."[1] The p53 protein is active when severe DNA damage is found in the cell. A double strand break, for example, constitutes serious damage and it must be repaired. When both strands of the DNA break,

---

1 Here, "p" stands for protein, "53" for the size of the protein — it is 53 kilodaltons (a unit of measure from protein chemistry). If the p53 gene is mutated, the protein p53 encoded by this gene can no longer perform its function. Yeast cells do not have a p53 gene, though, because their checkpoint mechanisms are much simpler. The nematode and the fruit fly do have the p53 gene; it is probably an important component of DNA damage checkpoints only in the case of multicellular organisms.

various proteins are recruited to the break site that were originally identified in yeast and which also exist in human cells.

One important protein that detects double strand breaks is the ATM protein. ATM stands for the grave, rare hereditary disease Ataxia telangiectasia (abbreviated AT), when it is mutated. There are two specific abnormalities in children having a mutation in the *ATM* gene: an unsteady gait (ataxia) and dilated arteries (telangiectasia). Patients start to show signs of developmental disorders by the age of two to three years. Their immune system is weak and often they develop cancer. AT is also regarded as a premature aging syndrome, because it causes a breakdown of the nervous system, neurodegeneration.

The cells of AT patients are extremely sensitive in reacting to ionizing radiation. This radiation leads to double strand breaks in the DNA that the cells cannot react to adequately due to the mutation in the *ATM* gene. AT patients are another example showing how errors in DNA repair processes can accelerate the aging process as well as lead to cancer development.

If a DNA strand breaks, the ATM protein binds to a loose end of the double helix of the DNA. The ATM sends an alarm signal to alert the cell: the DNA is severely damaged. The most important call for help goes to the p53 protein, which then sets off the highly complex sequence of the DNA damage response. On the one hand, p53 acts as a brake on the cell cycle — the cell must under no circumstance divide and reproduce as long as a chromosome is broken — by activating the same mechanisms that Hartwell and Weinert had already observed in yeast. But p53 can cripple far more than the process of cell division.

The cell cycle is then interrupted temporarily if there is a good chance that the damage can be repaired. If the damage is too great, however, p53 can drive the cell into senescence (from *senescere*, the Latin word for "aging"). This is precisely what Leonard Hayflick had observed in the cells he cultured in the 1960s. After a certain number of cell divisions, the cells eventually completely stopped growing. Once a cell enters into senescence, it does not just stop its division activity temporarily but terminates it entirely.

As a third option, p53 can also drive the cell to suicide or "programmed death." In this context, the suicide is known as apoptosis (from the Greek for "falling off"). Senescence and apoptosis can also be used as an expression of altruistic behavior of cells as part of an organism, in other words, self-sacrifice for the good of the larger unit. It had long been considered the height of absurdity to believe that cells should be able to kill themselves. As often happens in gerontology research, a revolution in thinking came once again from the humble nematode. Robert Horwitz, one of the pioneers of roundworm genetics, examined how the worms developed from the embryo up to the larva. It dawned on him that cells were born but died again even before the worm was mature. But the key point was that Horvitz identified a mutant in which the cells were not dying off during development. He called this and other similar mutants CED, as in "Cell Death abnormality." He noted that in the *ced-9* mutant, the CED-9 protein never stopped being active. CED-9 can therefore prevent cells from killing themselves off and make them go on living instead. In the *ced-9* mutants, cells were still present in the adult worm which should have died during the worm's development. Horvitz provided evidence that the suicide of a cell, apoptosis, was a genetically programmed process.

A fascinating question comes up here for biologists: what significance could this programmed cell death have for us humans? For this, Horvitz's discovery of the *ced-9* gene was the crucial bridge between worm research and human disease. The human equivalent of the nematode's CED-9 is the Bcl2 protein [37]. The protein was named b-c-l because cancerous blood cells in B-cell lymphomas produce massive amounts of the Bcl2 protein. The significance of this finding was overwhelming and caused a sea change in our thinking about cancer cells. CED-9 in the nematode and Bcl2 in humans prevent the self-destruction of the cell. Cells have a "cell death apparatus," which is kept at bay until the cell is supposed to commit suicide. This apparatus is turned off in the roundworm by the CED-9, and in humans by the Bcl2 protein. However, if p53 is active, a protein is produced which removes CED-9 or Bcl2 from the cell death apparatus thus unleashing it — and the cell dies. Now it was all clear: cancer cells fail to kill themselves because they have a malfunction in the apoptosis process. In the presence of Bcl2 overproduction, the lymphoma cells turn off their cell-death apparatus once and for all.

Mutations in the *p53* gene are even more serious than Bcl2 overproduction, because here not only the cell death apparatus but the entire checkpoint is disturbed. Thus, *p53* mutations also frequently lead to cancer formation — about half of all cancers have a mutation in *p53*. Much has been speculated about why a single gene, such as *p53*, is so central to the prevention of cancer. We already found the answer to this question in our review of evolutionary biology: *p53* mutations usually lead to cancer development only in advanced age. In our history of evolution, we were able to live well enough to have adequate cancer protection in our early years. Whether we were still well-protected from cancer after turning thirty (traditionally, humans had already procreated by then) was simply irrelevant.

Suppose we had a "better" p53; could that protect us against cancer? The answer was found once again using a model system. In the area of cancer research, the mouse is the most important animal model. Cancer can only occur in animals that consist of many cells. Many of the genes that are crucial for the onset of cancer are already present in the baker's yeast. Even in yeast, these genes function in the same way; they control the response to DNA damage and cell division. In nematodes, too, the same genes and the p53 protein control the programmed cell death as they do in humans, as I found out myself while working on my doctoral thesis. But neither yeast nor roundworms develop cancer. Although flies can develop "tumors" if their cell growth continues out of control, true cancer can only be induced in higher animals. Laboratory mice often die of cancer, as do humans. Let us remember, mice in the wild survive only about three-quarters of a year, until the winter cold does them in. In a protected environment, however, they can live for two to three years, thus reaching an age that never played a role in the evolution of the mouse. That being the case, aging laboratory mice do not have protection against age-related complications.

In mice, the development of cancer can be reproduced very accurately. Studies in mice have been (and still are) crucial to understanding cancer development. The same mutations that lead to the development of cancer in humans also cause cancer cells to develop in mice. That is why it is so important to conduct studies on mice when trying to develop therapies that can fight cancer in humans.

Whenever a new or improved drug against cancer is being developed, it is first tested in mice. The initial test evaluates whether a drug is not too toxic. Then, its effectiveness for fighting the cancer in the mouse is assessed. Until then, it would be unthinkable to consider testing a new drug in humans. A mouse with a mutation in the *p53* gene develops a variety of cancerous tumors quite similar to the one people get, when they are born with a mutation in their *p53* gene. Such Li-Fraumeni Syndrome patients are particularly vulnerable to cancer. However, Li-Fraumeni is a rare hereditary disease.

Most tumors develop when a spontaneous, unforeseen mutation occurs in the *p53* gene. Such spontaneous mutations can be caused when the DNA is damaged by, for example, tobacco smoke. Cancer cells carrying *p53* mutations are also very difficult to treat. This is due to the way in which cancer is treated nowadays. We will deal with cancer therapy itself in a later chapter, since it plays a very important role in the prospect of developing therapies for age-related diseases.

Mice whose *p53* gene is not working will develop cancer. What about mice whose p53 is more active than normal? Various mouse models have been developed to examine this question. Super-active p53 was produced in mice in two different ways [38], [39]. In these mice, p53 exceeded its normal functions and it drove more cells than usual into cell cycle arrest, senescence, and apoptosis. As you might already suspect, these mice were particularly well protected against cancer. Instead of developing tumors, the mice showed a very different disease: they were getting old at a very early age! The mice suffered from growth disturbances and showed early signs of aging. A hyperactive p53 can, in fact, protect against cancer, but it prevents cells from accomplishing their normal divisions. Consequently, the animals failed not only to grow up properly but also to renew and maintain their tissues, thus causing the body to age in an untimely way. So now it is also clear why we have the p53 that we have, and not a "better" one: more p53 activity can have dramatic negative effects.

With the example of too little and too much p53, we can draw some very basic conclusions about which mechanisms control the aging process. If a cell cannot respond to DNA damage with functioning checkpoints, it can lead to cancer because cells will continue to grow and multiply even though they should not. When inactive checkpoints allow cells to divide despite DNA damage, the result is mutation and uncontrolled cell growth.

Hyperactive p53, on the other hand, also disables the normal process of cell growth and causes cells to die that are needed for the functioning of the tissues. The organs and tissues are compromised in their function. Tissues can no longer be renewed because the stem cells, which are needed in order to replace cells in tissues such as skin, intestine, blood and others, cannot divide. The p53 protein has put the brakes on the cell cycle. When p53 is even more potent, cells die because they are driven into apoptosis, cell death. This leads to the loss of cells and thus the breakdown of tissues. This degradation is, in effect, aging: tissues lose their integrity and functionality, and they are less and less able to repair themselves with new cells.

Something similar happens to the body when DNA damage cannot be repaired. Persistent damage will activate p53 and the entire checkpoint apparatus. This brings the same results as in the mice with hyperactive p53: stem cells no longer divide, and the cells of the tissue die without being able to generate replacement cells.

If, on the other hand, the checkpoints are defective, DNA damage leads to mutations and abnormal chromosomes; and cancer will develop. Both cancer and premature aging can result from defective DNA repair mechanisms.

Interestingly, Spanish biologist Manuel Serrano has succeeded in producing a mouse that carries only one extra copy of the *p53* gene. In these animals, p53 functioned quite normally as opposed to the two aforementioned mice in which p53 was hyperactive. Serrano called this mouse "super p53," and in fact the extra copy of the *p53* gene did protect the mouse against cancer better than normal mice [40]. But the p53 was not so active that it inhibited tissue function or growth. This allowed the mouse to live a normal life, while it was also protected against cancer.

A little later Serrano's research group in Madrid even succeeded in producing a mouse that had extra copies of other anti-cancer genes [41] in addition to "super p53." These mice also remained immune to cancer and then lived longer than normal mice, presumably because they were so well protected from cancer. Thus it is possible, at least in mice, to improve cancer protection without accelerating the aging process. This principle could open up completely new avenues in medicine through improved checkpoint function.

Checkpoints and DNA repair are the body's natural mechanisms for preventing the onset of cancer and for maintaining the body's functions. DNA repair is the body's natural anti-aging mechanism. How do the highly complex DNA repair mechanisms of our cells work?

III.3 DNA repair: between aging and cancer development

It's time for genetic arts and crafts, with Angelina Jolie! Today we're building an enhanced immune system, or starting an arms race with our worst enemies: disease-causing agents, or pathogens. For this project we need to cut up the DNA, straighten it out and glue it together again. As we do this, we'll learn the dangers of acting hastily — and the benefits of doing a thorough repair vs. a fast but often negligent procedure. We'll also find out about the problems that damaged tools can cause.

As different as the causes of DNA damage may be, so are the changes in the DNA. The ultraviolet component of sunlight reacts directly with the nucleotides — the basic building blocks of DNA. Reactive oxygen radicals can also interact directly with the nucleotides and thus alter their properties. Various chemical agents can bind directly to the DNA and make them unusable as genetic material.

A particularly dangerous type of attack on the DNA comes from the ionizing radiation caused by X-rays or nuclear decay (radioactivity). This radiation is capable of removing electrons from atoms or molecules; the physicists calls that "ionization"; thus the term ionizing radiation. The effects of ionizing radiation have been the focus of research across the globe since the 1960s. The world was introduced to the effects of ionizing radiation in August 1945, when the United Stated dropped two atomic bombs on the Japanese cities of Hiroshima and Nagasaki. Tens of thousands of people were killed. At the point closest to detonation, people's skin was burnt off their bodies. Further afield, people died of acute radiation poisoning. Aftereffects, however, continued to develop for decades, because the ionizing radiation had damaged the genomes of ten thousand survivors. As a result of this damage to their genes, a high risk of cancer lay sleeping in the cells of the surviving victims.

In the post-war period, the main focus was on military research, and once nuclear power was seen as an efficient energy source, research was also carried out on the biological consequences of ionizing radiation. Initially, such research was conducted for military purposes, and it was not until much later, after the academic world got involved, that it began to bear real fruit for civilian society. Ionizing radiation transmits a high amount of energy and leads to the formation of reactive oxygen, a chemical radical, in the smallest possible space. We say radical here because the ionized atoms react pretty much with everything around and thus they can alter the chemical structure of molecules. The radicals react directly with the DNA and can even cause breakages in the DNA double strand. As we have seen, such double-strand breaks are extremely dangerous to the cell. Therefore the cell has different ways to repair such breaks. Unfortunately, repairing these breaks sometimes presents new dangers.

The simplest way to repair a double-strand break is to join the two ends back together again as quickly as possible. This "end-joining" connection is used very frequently. First, proteins bind the DNA ends to give the cell a signal that one of its chromosomes is broken. The DNA strands are brought together and recombined by a ligase, DNA ligase IV (remember the proteins connecting the DNA? from Latin, ligare = "to tie or link").

Research groups led by Penny Jeggo and Patrick Concannon studied cells from four patients who suffered from severe growth disorders and whose immune systems were not working [42]. Cells from the patients showed very typical signs of problems with the repair of DNA double-strand breaks. The cells were extremely sensitive to ionizing radiation. The patients looked suspiciously similar to people suffering from Ataxia telangiectasia who we encountered in the previous chapter. But none of the four patients showed any changes in the *ATM* gene. It was only when Jeggo and Concannon specifically looked into the patient cells' ability to connect the ends of double-strand breaks that they realized that the cells could not perform this repair. And indeed, in all four patients the researchers found a mutation in the gene encoding the *ligase IV*; consequently this premature aging syndrome was called ligase IV, or Lig4 syndrome for short.

Lig4 syndrome illustrates some particularly interesting aspects of the operation of double-strand break repair. The "end-joining" repair is a quick way to patch together double-strand breaks. It also has a very important function in our immune system.

The immune system has to protect the body from the dangerous effects of all possible infections. Viruses, bacteria and fungi constantly attack our cells.

Our infectious enemies come in different forms that are so versatile that they can penetrate the body and cause disease. Our immune system must constantly fend them off. Just as it is in humans, the genetic information of viruses and bacteria is also contained in their genome; only the genome of viruses is tiny compared to ours, and it often consists of just a few genes. The genomes of viruses and bacteria can be mutated just like ours, but they change much faster. Viruses are not much more than genes, encoded either as DNA or RNA, surrounded by a protective envelope and a few other protein structures that allow the virus to introduce its genetic information into our cells. In order to copy and read their genes, they basically use the machinery of our cells — viruses are therefore in every respect parasites through and through. They use the production machinery of our own cells to crank out viral proteins. Viruses program the cells in such a way that they are turned into mass production sites for viruses.

Eckard Wimmer, an American virologist and biochemist of German origin, set out in 2002 to prove that viruses are not living creatures but merely chemical structures. He decided to fabricate polioviruses completely synthetically. The Wimmer Group introduced into cells all the genetic information that is normally contained in the RNA genome of the poliovirus, by means of synthetically produced DNA. This genetic information of the virus succeeded in converting the cell to a poliovirus production plant. Wimmer's publication — just the year after the attacks on the World Trade Center — generated a sharp-tongued discussion about whether terrorists now had a guide to biological warfare through viruses, as well. Once in the cell, the small genomes of viruses multiply rapidly. At this high rate of duplication, many errors arise in the genomes of the viruses; in other words, they experience mutations. Viruses whose genome consists of RNA rather than DNA develop far more mutations. The human immunodeficiency virus (HIV) is particularly tricky because it mutates so fast that it can no longer be recognized by the immune system. This, on the other hand, makes biological warfare — whether by terrorists or military forces — quite impractical, because even the perpetrators may not be able to protect themselves against an ever changing and adapting virus.

Bacteria can also change their structure. The transfer of genes between different bacterial strains is especially dangerous. For example, resistance to an antibiotic can be transferred from a harmless to a dangerous strain of bacteria. The spread of resistance to antibiotics through genetic transfer and mutations is currently developing into an enormous worldwide health risk, also driven by unnecessary and uncontrolled use of antibiotics in humans and above all in livestock.

Our immune system is engaged in a constant battle against pathogens that can change their appearance quickly and thus are extremely adaptable. Above all, detecting them is the greatest challenge faced by our immune system. Two different systems are responsible for our immune defense: innate immunity and acquired, or adaptive, immunity. An innate immunity was formed way back in the early history of evolution; it allows even individual cells to defend against external attacks. The adaptive immune system can learn to identify pathogens and then direct the immune response to the dangerous pathogen. The adaptive immune response is taken over by specialized immune cells such as the B and T cells. These cells produce receptors. We already know about receptors as the proteins that sit on the surface of cells and recognize messengers, then send instructions to the cells' interior. Immune cells use special receptors with which they can recognize parts of pathogens instead of messenger substances. The B-cell receptors (BCR for short) and T-cell receptors (TCR) can distinguish a protein that originates from a virus, for example, from all other proteins that are found in a normal cell of the body.

For every pathogen, a specific receptor must now be formed. The information on the formation of the receptors must therefore be stored in the DNA encoding the receptors. A huge variety of BCRs and TCRs must reside in the genome of the B and T cells. The immune cells have to produce genetic information in order to be able to form specific BCRs and TCRs. To do that, the B and T cells have to alter the genes encoding these receptors in such a way that different receptors can be formed, which are then perfected so that they can clearly recognize a pathogen. The immune cells alter their genome in the section in which their DNA encodes the BCR or the TCR.

In order to be able to build a precise receptor, the cell has to take a hand to its own genome. Immune cells slice up their own DNA at very specific intervals and reassemble them in a different sequence. Thus, each BCR and TCR is different from every other one. For these receptors, there are approximately three hundred gene sections from which different parts can be lined up. The cutting of the DNA results in a double-strand break, only this break, in contrast to the ones caused by ionizing radiation, is targeted by specialized proteins called nucleases.

And then, the ends of the DNA that was cut have to be connected again. This means that this repair system also reconnects the ends of double-strand breaks. However, if patients have a mutation in the "end-joining" repair system, their B and T cells can no longer produce the receptors to recognize the disease agents. This is precisely why the immune system of LIG4 patients doesn't work. DNA repair is therefore important not only to defend against attacks on the genome, but also for pathogens such as bacteria and viruses.

When connecting the DNA ends back together, however, things can go wrong. This type of DNA repair is designed to patch together broken ends as quickly as possible and, just like a quick car repair job, there's often some fudging involved. When the gene portion of the B-cell receptor is restored, the wrong sections of the genome may be linked. Such erroneous connections of genome sections can have dramatic consequences. A gene with important and high-precision features, such as the regulation of cell division, can get completely out of whack. For example, the part of the BCR gene that normally regulates the gene activity could get linked to a section of a different gene, such as the MYC gene; then the B-cell will produce as much MYC protein as it was supposed to produce of the BCR. But the MYC gene encodes a transcription factor (and transcription factors, like the DAF-16 we talked about in the nematode worms, determine gene expression, i.e., how much of a gene is read). The MYC transcription factor, in turn, regulates the activity of genes that perform cell division. MYC determines how often a cell divides. High MYC production leads to the uncontrolled division of these B cells; the cells become cancer cells, and the person develops B-cell lymphoma.

Luckily, faulty links between sections of DNA with such tragic consequences are rare, and most of these errors pass without any consequences at all. This is due to the fact that only a small part of our chromosomes encode genes, while long stretches of DNA contain no genes at all. Consequently, errors in connecting DNA breaks often go entirely without consequences.

Unlike the specific type of double-strand breakage caused by the DNA-cutting nucleases during the formation of the BCR, double-strand breaks caused by exposure to ionizing radiation crop up randomly, somewhere in the genome; the probability of a gene being struck is very low. Therefore, the cell most often simply joins the DNA ends. A wrong linkage between a very active gene, like the BCR gene, and a gene like MYC, is very rare — but it can lead to the development of cancer nevertheless; that is due to the fact that the cell now divides far too frequently and produces many cells that constantly pump out the MYC transcription factor.

However, the cell also has a highly accurate repair mechanism for double-strand breaks. The so-called "recombination repair" uses an undamaged copy of the damaged genome section. It then combines undamaged DNA so that the broken DNA can be replaced. Obviously, this type of repair requires an undamaged copy, so the recombination repair is applied only when the genome is being duplicated. This is the case after the DNA has been replicated but the cell has not yet split in two.[1] During the recombination repair, the same sequence that was in place where the double-strand break occurred (the sequence of the nucleotides that determine the genetic information) is searched for in the undamaged copy of the affected chromosome. If this section is found, the part of the DNA around the fragment is removed, and the DNA sequence is restored using a copy of the undamaged chromosome as a template.

The highly complex recombination repair takes much more time than the simple re-linking of breaks. Therefore many processes, especially cell division, have to be adjusted around the repair process. Ataxia telangiectasia patients cannot perform the recombination repair because their *ATM* gene is not working. The ATM protein, together with a whole arsenal of specialized recombination proteins, binds to a double-strand break and coordinates the checkpoint response during which the recombination machinery searches for the undamaged DNA sequence. Ataxia telangiectasia patients suffer from both premature aging and, often, from early blood cancer too, because the DNA repair cannot be performed properly.

Another important genetic defect, which leads to errors in the recombination repair is located in the *BRCA1* gene. This gene gained fame after Angelina Jolie made it public that she carried a mutation of her own *BRCA1* gene. Two of the genes associated with "Breast Cancer," *BRCA1* and *BRCA2*, were discovered in cancer patients. Anyone who has a mutation in one of these genes carries a high risk of developing cancer of the breast or ovaries. Women whose family members have had breast cancer or ovarian cancer can, after extensive consultation with their gynecologist, decide to have both *BRCA* genes sequenced in order to find out whether they are carrying a mutation in these genes. When Ms. Jolie was found to have a mutation in the *BRCA1* gene, she decided to have precautionary surgery to remove the breast tissue before any cancer could develop. Such a step is certainly drastic and should be considered carefully. Breast cancer is highly dangerous and avoidance is the only safe strategy, especially if you are in an extremely high-risk category such as carriers of the *BRCA* mutations. The two BRCA proteins are directly involved in recombination repair. Without them, this repair process does not work and there will be errors in the repair of double-strand breaks. This allows wrong connections to be made between chromosomes, which then create errors in the way cell growth is regulated. This leads to uncontrolled cell division culminating in the development of cancer.

---

1 Some cell types, such as human eggs, can remain in such an intermediate phase of the cell cycle for decades and they can accurately repair any damage using the recombination repair mechanism.

As to why the BRCA gene defects lead so specifically to breast and ovarian cancer is not really understood. With respect to breast cancer, for example, metabolic by-products of the female sex hormone estrogen can even damage the DNA, whereas in white blood cells double-strand breaks may show up naturally during maturation in B- and T-cells of the BCR and TCR genes.

Both types of double-strand break repair have advantages and disadvantages: accurate recombination repair is time-consuming, but the fast repair is prone to error. Interestingly, cells still have a "backup" option to somehow repair double-strand breaks even if neither the end-joining nor recombination works. This could lead to faulty repair and thus to mutations, which in turn can cause cancer to develop.

III.4 DNA damage causes cancer

Now we'll see what Boveri learned from sea urchins and why we must never feed rabbits with coal tar. You will also get to know what carcinogens are creeping into our DNA and preventing it from performing its tasks properly. Poor linkages like these, as well as bad copies, cause cancer.

Even before it was linked to the aging process, DNA damage was known as a primary cause of cancer. The German biologist Theodor Boveri first recognized the fact that cancer is a disease of the chromosomes in the early 20th century. To prove that hereditary information has to be contained in the nucleus of the cell, Boveri extracted cell nuclei from the eggs of sea urchins and then fertilized them with several sperm cells. Using microscopic research on cell nuclei, Boveri came to the conclusion that the chromosomes in the cell nuclei are the actual carriers of the genetic information. Based on the observations of pathologist David von Hansemann, who described the unequal number of chromosomes in cancerous tissue late in the 19th century, Boveri attributed the development of cancer to the unequal distribution of chromosomes to daughter cells, which is called *aneuploidy* [45]. Boveri's hypothesis could be considered the beginning of our understanding of what causes cancer. Today it is clear that aneuploidy is an important factor in cancer development. Especially after the checkpoints are inactivated — for example by mutations in the *p53* gene — aneuploidy can make the cancer cells even more aggressive.

The first references to what causes cancer to develop date back to the 19th century, when chimney sweeps were found to be affected by cancer of the scrotum. A few decades later, Japanese researchers Yamagiwa and Ichikawa observed that rabbits who had been administered coal tar were affected by cancer [46]. Later the critical chemical substance in the coal tar was identified that could cause skin cancer in mice.

Cancer-causing chemical substances, called carcinogens (once again borrowed from the Greek: karkinos for "cancer" and genesis for "production"), have a spatial structure that allows them to lie in the helix structure of the DNA and then chemically react with the DNA thus altering its structure.

After carcinogens have been identified, safety limits can be established and the risk of cancer can be reduced. That being said, cigarette smoke contains a large number of chemical carcinogens and it is the smoker who decides to expose himself to a high risk of cancer.

Chemical changes to the DNA building blocks, the nucleotides, can cause the DNA production to stall during copying, that is, during DNA replication. In addition, copying errors occur when the correct new nucleotide is not incorporated because the original has been chemically altered and therefore is not correctly recognized.

Mutations can also occur during normal replication. The replication machinery works very precisely in incorporating the correct nucleotides during the DNA copying process, but replication also has to take place very quickly. After all, the sequence of all three billion nucleotides has to be copied if the daughter cells are to get all the genetic information. To correct errors immediately after copying the DNA, the replication engine may do a quick patch-up and remove the wrong nucleotides from the fresh copy. In addition, during replication, the mismatch repair system also monitors whether the wrong nucleotides have been inserted.

Mutations in mismatch repair genes resulting in flawed repair proteins result in a higher error rate every time the DNA copy-operation takes place. This leads to a particularly high risk of developing colorectal cancer due to the very high division rates of cells in the bowel. Indeed, defects in mismatch repair underlie hereditary non-polypoid colorectal carcinoma (HNPCC).

III.5 The dangers of the sun's rays and the "Moon Children" phenomenon

Now to the enemy whom we cannot escape — nor would we want to: the Sun. Why is she not only friendly, but also deadly, and why is it that Moon Children can only meet her if they're dressed up like astronauts? And then, there's another gang of kids who do not get cancer and yet they are already dying at 12, and a few words about what is wrong with incorrect pair formations, illegible information and flawed interpretations during cancer development.

Cancer is a disease that can affect even children — just think of how many cases of leukemia strike the very young. However, cancer is mainly a disease that comes with aging. As we age, the risk of developing cancer increases dramatically.

As Boveri recognized long ago, cancer is a disease of the genes. The genetic defects that lead to cancer are sometimes inherited, as in Li-Fraumeni patients or women with hereditary breast or ovarian cancer, who carry mutations in the BRCA genes. In most cases, cancer patients acquired the genetic changes only in the course of life, mutations that then transform their own cells into cancer cells. As we have seen, these mutations can be caused by a variety of different carcinogens. The crucial factor that leads to cancer in our skin is the ultraviolet radiation from the sun. UV radiation causes particularly malicious DNA damage. Often it has to do with sunburns suffered earlier in life usually during childhood. Above all, sunbathing is extremely risky because it exposes the skin to very intense UV radiation — after all, we like to get a tan as quickly as possible. As vicious as cancer is, it only breaks out decades after the initial damage is done. Mutations can remain dormant for a long time without any visible effect. At first, we only notice the pleasant sunshine, the warmth. Vitamin D is produced; endorphins send happiness throughout the body. Our body needs the sunlight! But this is a life-threatening risk.

And again, as we already covered while discussing the evolutionary basis of aging: DNA damage and the mutations that come along with it only lead to cancer much later, when we are no longer equipped to keep the consequences at bay. So we sit down in the sun and feel good about it, not realizing that we are starting a chain of effects that will show up much later. The incidence of skin cancer is increasing dramatically. Every year, more than 5 million people are diagnosed with skin cancer in the United States. At particular danger are people who went to tanning salons during their teenage years and are now developing skin cancer twenty years later.

The reason why so much time passes from the first attack on the genome until ultimately cancer erupts is because it takes not only one but several mutations for a cell to become a cancer cell. In the late 1990s, American cancer researcher Robert Weinberg succeeded in transforming human cells into cancer cells by performing three genetic modifications [47]. This suggests that mutations in three genes are sufficient to induce cancer. What types of genes must these three be, that together they can cause such a dramatic disease as cancer? Weinberg first introduced the gene for telomerase into the cells. Telomerase is a protein that protects the ends of the chromosomes from shortening. Weinberg also took a gene named RAS that had been switched on permanently by a mutation and which constantly signaled to the cell that it should divide. In order to complete the trio of cancer genes, Weinberg's team added another gene called the large-T oncogene of a monkey virus (simian virus 40, or SV40) into the cells. The protein formed by this viral gene de-activates the well-known p53 protein in the cells and thus disrupts the checkpoints that would otherwise protect the cell from uncontrolled growth. Cancer specialists (oncologists) call genes that actively stimulate the growth of cancer cells oncogenes; *RAS* as well as *MYC*, which we talked about in connection with the B cells of the immune system, are typical oncogenes in the human genome. With these three genetic changes, normal human cells can become cancer cells.

Cancer cells that occur naturally in the human body often show hundreds of mutations and changes in the structure of the chromosomes, such as aneuploidy, that is, gain or loss of chromosomes, as Boveri discovered. The accumulation of so many genetic changes is due to the failure of checkpoints to respond to DNA damage. Hence, mutations continue to accumulate in the tumor cells during progression. It takes a very long time, however, to accumulate all the mutations that are necessary to transform a cell into a cancer cell. So even if UV radiation created the first critical mutation, additional mutations are required. Repeated sunbathing is precisely the kind of behavior that causes these additional mutations.

There are patients for whom even everyday sunshine is too much of a risk: colloquially, they are sometimes known as "Moon Children," since they have to stay out of the daylight entirely, so as not to develop skin cancer. Afflicted with Xeroderma pigmentosum (XP), these children first show inflammatory reactions and are covered with freckles, with extreme pigmentation of those parts of their skin that is exposed to sunlight. The children go on to develop deadly skin tumors. Moon children had a difficult life and often they spent their childhood isolated, because playing outdoors was a deadly risk.

Only in recent decades has DNA repair research succeeded in shedding light (in the truest sense of the word "light") not only on the cause of the disease, but also in the life of young patients. In the 1960s, James Cleaver examined cells from patients suffering from Xeroderma pigmentosum. He exposed these cells to UV radiation and gave them nucleotides, DNA building blocks that he had previously labeled radioactively. Thus, he could determine whether the nucleotides would be incorporated into the DNA of the cells by simply following the radioactivity in the cells' DNA. Normal cells incorporated the nucleotides into their DNA after UV irradiation. They did this because they repaired their UV-damaged DNA. The cells cut away the part of their DNA that contained the damage and filled the resulting gap with new nucleotides. When Cleaver carried out the same experiment with the cells of Moon children, he found that none of the labeled nucleotides were incorporated. Cleaver proved that the patients' cells could not repair their DNA after UV irradiation. Thus an explanation was found for the extremely high UV sensitivity of the patient cells. It was suddenly clear that the problem was the failure to repair the UV-induced DNA damage.

Although this disease cannot yet be cured, this breakthrough led to an effective means of preventing its worst excesses. If a child is diagnosed with Xeroderma pigmentosum today, the parents have a number of ways to minimize their child's suffering and above all the risk of cancer. The children must be protected from even small amounts of UV radiation. Because normal clothing allows too much UV radiation to pass through to the skin, they need special sun-block fabrics. NASA developed special clothing to protect astronauts who are exposed to extremely high UV radiation when their travels take them beyond the earth's protective atmosphere, which serves as a UV filter. If the "Moon Children" wear clothes made using the same technology, they can go outdoors during the day and play with their friends. The windows at home and at school have to be covered with UV-blocking film. UV measuring devices can give them an exact risk assessment before they leave the house, letting them know if the cloud cover is sufficient to trap a large part of the UV radiation.

However, there are some Xeroderma pigmentosum patients whose suffering is not limited to the skin alone. Patients are categorized in Groups A to G, depending on which of their genes is mutated. We know today that about thirty different proteins are involved in the repair of UV-induced DNA damage and it is very possible that even more factors await their discovery. So far, mutations in seven genes were found that can lead to this disease.

Patients with mutations in *XP* genes *A*, *B*, *D* and *G* also develop neurological disorders. In these patients, nerve cells die early. On the basis of these patients' disease patterns, the two effects of DNA damage become clear again: cancer formation and the degeneration of tissues, in this case brain tissues: a very typical sign of aging.

In the mid-1940s, the English pediatrician Edward Cockayne examined an extremely short-lived child whose nervous system had not developed properly and whose eyesight failed. Children who are diagnosed with this Cockayne Syndrome (CS) show initially no particular abnormalities as newborns, but already within the first few years of their short lives their body's growth is severely retarded. Soon thereafter, various tissues start to show signs of degeneration. Nerve cells die, and the patient's brain and ability to control movement are disturbed. Cockayne Syndrome patients typically die at the age of twelve, often due to arteriosclerosis and kidney failure. In very severe cases, death occurs as early as the age of six. Also the skin of Cockayne Syndrome patients reacts very sensitively to sunlight similarly to Xeroderma pigmentosum patients. In stark contrast to Xeroderma pigmentosum patients, however, they do not develop skin cancer.

The inherited mutations underlying Cockayne Syndrome affect two genes, the *CSA* and the *CSB* gene. The proteins encoded by these two genes play a role in repairing DNA damage caused by UV light. However, the disease patterns caused by mutations in the XP genes or mutations in the CS genes are completely different. XP mutations lead to skin cancer, whereas CS mutations lead to growth disorders and tissue degeneration in many organs and tissue: degradation that is so typical of aging. This is why Cockayne Syndrome is also referred to as *progeria*, a disease that leads to premature aging.

So far we have learned of many genetic diseases in which patients who carry mutations in genes that are necessary for DNA repair suffer from premature aging and develop cancer. However, the examples of Xeroderma pigmentosum and Cockayne Syndrome teach us that malfunction in DNA repair may lead either to cancer or to premature aging. Therefore, these diseases are very important to our understanding of how DNA damage triggers aging.

The *XP* and *CS* genes are part of one of the most complex DNA repair machineries, so-called *nucleotide excision repair*, NER for short. The name itself describes how the repair works. A piece of the damaged DNA strand is cut out, which is called "excision" (from the Latin *excidere* "to excise") of nucleotides. There are two reasons why NER is so complex and needs so many different repair factors. On the one hand, NER recognizes certain types of DNA damage that are not easy to detect because of their structure. On the other hand, not only the damaged nucleotide but a piece consisting of about 30 nucleotides must be excised from the DNA strand, and then this piece has to be re-built.

The NER machinery recognizes DNA damage that leads to changes in its spatial structure. Typical examples are the two changes that we have been discussing, and that are directly caused by the impact of UV rays on the DNA and lead to the direct chemical linkage of the bases of the nucleotides. The energy of the ultraviolet radiation then produces a direct connection of two adjacent T building blocks of the DNA. Such a chemical compound is called *cyclobutane pyrimidine dimer*, or CPD. Instead of the nucleotides being linked only by the backbone of the DNA, they are now directly linked to one another via the bases. This direct chemical connection leads to a small spatial change in the DNA structure. Although at first sight it is minor, the effects of such a change are dramatic — because it means that a gene can no longer be read. The transcription, i.e., the rewriting of the genes from the DNA to the mRNA during gene expression, comes to a standstill when a UV-induced CPD blocks the path.

The replication, i.e., the copying of the DNA strands, can ignore such damage. It can copy the strands — but not correctly. The replication machinery is not able to chemically interpret the bases that have been directly connected, in order to place them with the right bases in the new strand. Therefore, after UV radiation, mutations are generated during replication. Mutations, in turn, can lead to malfunctions of genes and can cause the development of cancer. DNA damage caused by UV radiation occurs directly when exposed to the sun without protection. That makes this kind of damage very frequent and extremely dangerous.

UV damage in the DNA can have two different consequences. On the one hand, it often triggers mutations if the damage is not repaired before the DNA is copied. On the other hand, it can also halt the process of gene expression, transcription. For these two consequences of UV damage, NER has two different damage detection mechanisms.

Problems with replication affect the whole genome, because the genome has to be copied in its entirety before a cell can divide. Cell divisions are always taking place in the skin, because our outer skin layer constantly has to be renewed. Here, NER proteins scan the entire genome after UV damage in a process called *global genome-NER*, or *GG-NER*. The XPC protein is always scanning the chromosomes for damage that alters the structure of the DNA. A mutation in the *XPC* gene means that this scanning is no longer performed. Any UV damage thus remains, and during replication can lead to mutations by faulty copying of the damaged DNA. Patients whose XPC protein is not working will develop Xeroderma pigmentosum, the form that exclusively affects the skin.

It is quite different during the reading — the transcription — of genes with UV damage in their sequence. Here the transcription stops, and *transcription-coupled-NER*, or *TC-NER*, begins. If damage is found while the transcription is paused, the CSB Protein Alarm sounds, and the CSA protein is called to launch the NER repair. However, if the CSA or CSB fails to function — as with Cockayne Syndrome patients — the transcription machinery stops where the damage cannot be repaired.

After the damage is detected, GG-NER and TC-NER use the same core NER machinery. The XPA, -B, -D and -G proteins are all part of this shared NER machinery. Consequently, patients who carry mutations in these genes also suffer from skin pathologies (strong pigmentation, dry skin, skin cancer), like XPC patients, and they have malfunctions and tissue degradation in the nervous system, too.

Defects in the TC-NER do not cause more mutations in the genome. Instead, they block transcription. However, if the replication machine comes upon a transcription unit that was left unrepaired, a collision may ensue. Now the replication is stuck. As a result, the cell is barely able to divide anymore, let alone transform itself into a cancer cell, because the DNA has to be copied every time before the cell can divide. But without even the necessary cell divisions that are required to build and renew tissues, tissues cannot grow, and cells will die when there is so much DNA damage that it leads to blockage.

This is followed by growth disturbances. The loss of cells means tissue degeneration — these patients age in fast-forward mode. In this case the accelerated aging is not caused by mutations resulting from DNA damage but rather by the unrepaired DNA damage itself. In contrast to DNA damage that was left unrepaired, mutations are often a result of a failed DNA repair attempt. The faulty repair allows the cell to continue to perform its function, but it carries the risk that mutations in genes responsible for checkpoints and cell growth can cause cancer.

How can damage in the DNA have such serious effects on the whole body? Once again, studies conducted on mice have been particularly enlightening.

In order to develop mouse models for rare hereditary diseases such as Xeroderma pigmentosum and Cockayne Syndrome, first you have to know which genes cause the disease, what mutation the patients inherited. The NER genes were already known in bacteria and yeast cells, but the first human DNA repair gene was identified by Jan Hoeijmakers and Dirk Bootsma, researchers in Rotterdam, only in the 1980s. This was not a simple undertaking. It helped to have cells from Chinese hamsters into which pieces of the human genome could be introduced particularly easily. A number of such hamster cells had already been identified, some of which were particularly sensitive to UV radiation. These cells — like the cells of the Xeroderma pigmentosum and Cockayne Syndrome patients — had malfunctions in the DNA repair genes. Hoeijmakers and Bootsma used these genetic defects in the hamster cells to test which parts of the human genome would restore the DNA repair in the UV-sensitive hamster cells. Because such genome sections, according to their logic, would contain exactly the genes necessary for the DNA repair. First, the two Dutchmen identified the NER gene *ERCC1*. This was followed by a series of other NER genes such as the XP and CS genes. From there, one could proceed and identify the mutations in exactly these genes in the patient. The critical repair genes had been found.

After that the process didn't take so long and modern methods were used to generate mice that contained exactly the same mutations as the patients. Using these mice, one could investigate the effects of DNA repair defects on cancer development, body growth and premature aging.

The mice that were made to mimic the mutation in the Cockayne Syndrome patients remained short-lived, and after only a few weeks they looked like mice that were at the end of their two- to three-year life span. In the most severe cases, the mice died three weeks after birth. Thus, an experimental animal model was found that enabled researchers to test the effects of a specific DNA repair defect.

And then a completely unexpected discovery was made: In Jan Hoeijmakers' laboratory, the Greek biologist George Garinis was trying to create a comprehensive picture of the expression, i.e., the use of all the genes in the prematurely aging mice. The mRNAs were then measured and compared with the mRNAs of normal mice of the same age.[1] Remember that the mRNA is created after the rewriting (transcription) of DNA into RNA, which is then transported from the nucleus to translate into proteins. After that, it is possible to infer which genes are particularly active — that is, which ones produce a large amount of mRNA — and which genes are inactive — those that produce very little or no mRNA at all. Once the gene activity or *gene expression* has been analyzed this way, one can determine which biological processes occur in a cell or in a tissue.

Garinis observed next that the mice with the same genetic defect as the Cockayne Syndrome patients showed an extremely low expression of those genes that use the insulin-like growth factor (termed *IGF-1* for short) to control the growth process [48], [49]. In fact, only small amounts of the growth factor IGF-1 were measured in the entire body of the mouse. Now we remember that decreased IGF-1 activity, whether due to Kopchick's mutation in the growth hormone receptor (the GH receptor) or in the Snell and Ames dwarf mice, leads to reduced body growth, just as it does in the short-lived Cockayne Syndrome mice. But unlike the Cockayne Syndrome mice, which died early, the Ames and Snell dwarf mice or Kopchick's mice, which lack the receptor for sensing the growth hormone, are long-lived. Then, together with Garinis, we systematically looked at the similarities between the mice that were degenerating prematurely and those that were long-lived. And indeed, the two extremes — premature aging and retarded aging — turned out to be strikingly similar [50].

The key question that remained was: How is DNA damage causing premature aging linked to reduced IGF-1 activity, which prolongs life in animals from the nematode to the mammal? For this purpose, we had at hand the ideal experimental system for testing the different effects of gene defects in cells of Xeroderma pigmentosum and Cockayne Syndrome patients. With the distinct outcomes of those two DNA repair defects we were able to study which DNA damage responses cause premature aging and which ones, on the contrary, lead to the uninterrupted growth of cells

---

1 Ideally, one would of course measure the quantity of proteins, but proteins are much more difficult to measure than mRNAs. Even nowadays, with the huge advances made in measuring proteins, it is still not possible to measure a cell or a tissue with the same sensitivity and accuracy. However, measuring the amount of all the mRNAs does not pose particular difficulties.

as cancer cells. We noted that only those specific forms of DNA damage that halted the transcription reduced the IGF-1 activity [51]. If this damage persists, the expression of the genes that encode the IGF-1 receptors and the growth hormone GH is diminished; both growth factors are then missing so they cannot stimulate the cells in the body to go into cell division, and the growth of the tissues stops. The reduced activity of these two receptors is also decisive in making for an extended life.

How does this damage-response program work? Can it help the body deal with damage in the DNA? To answer this question, we in Cologne, Germany, turned once again to the simple nematode. Roundworms that carry mutations in the *CSA* or *CSB* genes are sensitive to UV radiation and their bodies completely stop growing. Also, the worms activate the same program as the Cockayne syndrome mice: The crucial protein that allows the worms to live longer, DAF-16, is activated when it is switched on due to reduced IGF-1 signals (in the worm, this is *daf-2*). In our studies, we have found that vigorous DAF-16 activity allows the roundworms to continue growing even if they cannot repair DNA damage at all [52]. The tissues of adult worms continue to function as long as DAF-16 is active. Thanks to DAF-16 the worms can survive, even if the DNA in the genome remains damaged. The "longevity program" controlled by DAF-16 allows the animal to tolerate persistent DNA damage and to live a fairly long life through damage tolerance. However, with advancing age, the ability of DAF-16 to respond declines. Old worms no longer activate DAF-16 and instead succumb to the accumulated DNA damage.

These results show a fascinating link between DNA damage and the genetic mechanisms that extend life: cells react by blocking off the consequences of DNA damage with a "longevity" program that can maintain the function of tissues and organs. This program, which is run by DAF-16, protects cells and tissues against stress and their function is improved, the same as in long-lived animals.

In contrast to worms, the tissues of mice and humans need continuous cell divisions not only for their growth but also for their maintenance. Here, the diminished activity of the IGF-1 signaling pathway results in reduced body growth. The advantage of reducing the growth signals is that it prevents cancer. Just so, Cockayne Syndrome patients are indeed well protected from cancer. Thus, the longevity program can counteract the adverse effects of DNA damage. This is apparently the case not only in prematurely aging patients but also during our normal aging.

III.6. DNA damage responses in aging

Everything in its own time: why is growth necessary in the spring of life and dangerous in the autumn, why does the body we inhabit need so much renewal, and why is it that this can only take place in a limited fashion in old age?

When we investigated the gene expression of prematurely aging mice, we also found that they are astonishingly similar to those of mice in the waning days of their lives. The naturally aged mice also showed low expression of the genes involved in the IGF-1 signaling pathway. As in the mouse, smaller amounts of growth factors are produced in humans with increasing age, and also less IGF-1.

After all what we have learned from model systems, from the *daf-2* nematodes to the long-lived dwarf mice, we can conclude that a reduction of growth serves to preserve life. In mice and humans, the deprivation of growth factors also has the consequence of reducing the risk of cancer. Cancer cells cannot grow by themselves; they need growth hormones from the body. This is the reason why tumors may develop when we are older, but they grow slowly. Conversely, the cells of child blood cancer patients proliferate rapidly.

But in humans the diminished production of growth messengers also has a completely different side. It may decrease hormone production, even reducing the growth hormone itself, and can lead to bone loss. Osteoporosis in women develops gradually after menopause. For a long time people tried using hormone therapies to counter the negative effects of the decreasing hormone production that comes with aging. However, in line with what we have learned about cancer formation and the growth of cancer cells, such treatment always entails an increased risk of cancer. These pros and cons must be carefully considered before deciding on any hormone therapy. We will learn more about this in the chapter on aging therapies.

Anyway, cell growth is at the foundation not only of the diseased growth of cancer, but also for the growth and maintenance necessary for the normal function of many tissues.

The mouse model of the Hutchinson-Gilford-Progeria Syndrome (HGPS) also stays behind in body growth, much like HGPS patients. When the Spanish researcher Carlos López-Otín learned about the research results from Rotterdam, he examined the IGF-1 values in his HGPS mice. These prematurely aging mice also showed reduced amounts of IGF-1 in their bloodstream, quite similar to the Cockayne Syndrome mice. When López-Otín injected his mice with IGF-1, they grew again and were able to develop [53]. This made it clear that the program that should protect the aging body from the effects of DNA damage by reducing cell and tissue growth also prevents the growth that is essential during the early stages of life and can lead to severe developmental disorders.

The HGPS and Cockayne syndrome mice, therefore, in principle use the right program to ward off the increasing instability of their genomes, but they do so at a life stage where this is completely inappropriate and then the negative effects clearly outweigh the benefits.

One tissue that requires constant renewal is the blood system. White and red blood cells must always be produced. While we in Rotterdam were studying the impact of blocking DNA damage, Raul Mostoslavsky and Fred Alt were in Boston, studying a mouse that also aged dramatically fast. This mouse had a mutation in the *Sirtuin 6* gene and was highly sensitive to DNA damage.

The Sirt6 mouse also showed errors in the formation of white blood cells. Surprisingly, this failure did not extend to the stem cells of the blood itself. The stem cells formed completely normal white blood cells, if they were transplanted into normal mice. But even stem cells from normal mice, transplanted into the Sirt6 mice, could not generate a significant quantity of white blood cells [54]. The mice lacking Sirtuin 6 had too little of the IGF-1 growth factor in their blood system. These results suggested that the small amounts of growth factors were insufficient to enable the stem cells to divide, for example the stem cells that should have been producing white blood cells, thereby the regeneration, or renewal, of tissues was impeded.

A similar finding was made by the German physician scientist Lenhard Rudolph. He was conducting studies on mice that prematurely aged because their telomeres, i.e., the structures protecting the ends of the chromosomes, were too short [55]. The mice could not produce enough white blood cells from their blood stem cells. The blood stem cells themselves functioned perfectly in normal mice, but even normal blood stem cells with intact telomeres could not form white blood cells in the mice with shortened telomeres.

Here, another negative effect caused by decreasing growth factors in old age is played out: the capacity of the stem cells to regenerate decreases as we age. Growth factors are essential to stem cells so they can divide and to form new cells. So there are no simple answers to the question what is the perfect balance for an aging body.

On tissues that are already developed, reduced IGF-1 activity has a positive effect. Therefore, the *daf-2* mutation, which inactivates the IGF-1 receptor in the nematode worms and then leads to the activation of DAF-16, is almost completely positive. All the tissues in the adult nematodes are completely formed. Aside from the germ line, no cells are dividing. In the nematode, the somatic tissues, i.e., the body (in contrast to the germ cells) have no stem cells and are not regenerated. They don't need to, during the two-to-three weeks' life of the nematode.

There are also human tissues that are formed once and never regenerate. Our nerve cells, for example, are formed during our early development and have to serve us all our lives. If a nerve cell dies, it cannot be replaced. Therefore the degradation, the degeneration, of nerve cells is irreversible in old age.

Even so, stem cells were found some years ago in the brains of mice and humans. But this is probably mainly a relic from our evolutionary history. These cells form new nerve cells only to a very limited extent, apparently even less in humans than in the mouse. Almost all of our nerve cells are irreplaceable. Also the nerve cells that are responsible for our cognitive abilities cannot be renewed. If they die, they are lost forever. Therefore, dementia is a central challenge for aging humanity.

III.7. Dementia: When our nerves are old

Advanced age is the time when the nerve cells fold up their tents and move away. Some things, such as memory or the ability to eat and to cope with everyday life, are lost. Doctors speak of Alzheimer's disease and Parkinson's disease. These are due to deposits of toxic protein compounds in the brain and to genes that are overwhelmed in their task of resupplying the nervous system.

We have already seen that prematurely aging patients very often suffer from a degeneration of nerve cells. The most obvious consequences would be an unsteady gait, a loss of motor control and coordination. The declining motor skills can be caused, for example, by the death of the so-called *Purkinje cells*, which coordinate motor function from the cerebellum. One consequence is a disorder in the course of movement — also called *ataxia* — a clear sign of premature aging in Ataxia telangiectasia patients. Those who are affected make too large or wide movements past the target, or they can only stand upright or sit straight with a support.

DNA repair defects, such as those that cause Cockayne Syndrome, lead to the breakdown of nerve cells, which in turn leads to severe cognitive loss.

Even in natural aging, neurodegenerative diseases arise, that is, problems caused by deterioration of the nervous system. It is estimated that nearly half of all people suffer from dementia after the age of eighty-five. This is a frightening number. It means that almost every second person, if he reaches a certain age, has to anticipate the loss of cognitive performance. It is already clear that this affects all the individual families involved but it also represents an overwhelming burden for society as a whole. There is also a growing debate about whether with the use of terms like "dementia" amounts to premature stigmatization. As long as there is no cure, people with dementia are a normal part of our modern aging society.

The most common neurodegenerative disease is Alzheimer's disease, which accounts for about 60 percent of dementia cases. This is followed by the far less common Parkinson's a disease, which is characterized by tremors. At the turn of the 20th century, Alois Alzheimer described the illness now named after him and which is about to become the scourge of our aging society in the 21st century. Alzheimer examined the fifty-year-old Auguste Deter in the Psychiatric Clinic of Frankfurt in Germany and dubbed the illness "pre-senile dementia" [56].

People with Alzheimer's disease gradually lose their cognitive abilities and develop conspicuous behavioral problems. As the disease progresses, they lose their ability to remember and often can no longer recognize close relatives. The day-to-day routine is lost, patients cannot carry out the simplest things, even eating can be difficult. Alzheimer's disease is a particularly insidious disease because it creeps up gradually and affects the entire social environment.

After Auguste Deter's death, Alois Alzheimer was able to have the deceased patient's brain sent to Munich, where he had become a laboratory director. Alzheimer's patients' brains have characteristic senile plaques and fibrils, that is, fine fibers. The plaques, as we now know, consist of aggregates of what are called *beta-amyloid peptides*. The fibrils, on the other hand, are formed in the interior of the cell by the *tau* protein. These are the defining characteristics of the brain of an Alzheimer's patient. In fact, the disease actually seems to be caused by a variant of the beta-amyloid peptide ("peptide" is a term for proteins which are relatively short), which consists of 42 amino acids. These peptides are derived from the *amyloid precursor protein* (APP).[1] The beta-amyloid-42 peptide is considered to be toxic because it forms smaller aggregates (*oligomers*) or larger aggregates (*polymers*) in combination with some other beta-amyloid peptides. The polymers then form the typical beta-amyloid or senile plaques. Although these plaques are considered to be markers of the Alzheimer's disease-stricken brain, it appears that it is not so much these frightening plaques but rather the smaller beta-amyloid oligomers that are responsible for the disease. In patients who develop Alzheimer's disease early on, mutations in two *presenilin* genes have been found. Presenilin 1 and 2 form part of the *gamma secretase*, the critical enzyme responsible for producing the beta-amyloid-42 peptide. In addition,

---

1 Beta-amyloid is produced when the amyloid precursor protein (APP) is divided at specific places. APP can be cleaved, or divided, by alpha-secretase or successively by beta-secretase and gamma-secretase. These enzymes cleave APP at very specific locations. As a product of gamma secretase, the beta-amyloid peptide is formed as either a 40- or 42-amino acid-long peptide.

changes in the *APP* gene have also been identified. An analysis of Auguste Deter's DNA in 2013 revealed that it contained a mutation in the presenilin 1 gene [57].

In contrast to Deter's disease, the most common form of Alzheimer's disease occurs only at an advanced age. For this late-onset form of Alzheimer's disease, a certain form of *apolipoprotein E* (ApoE) was discovered in 1993 as a genetic risk factor [58], [59]. The *ApoE* gene occurs in humans in different variants; which variant we carry in our genome determines how high our personal risk is of developing Alzheimer's disease. The type 4 variant of the *ApoE* gene is found very frequently in Alzheimer patients. If the Alzheimer's risk of an eighty-four-year-old is normally about 20%, the rate is 50% among those who have the *ApoE4* variant in just one of the two *ApoE* genes. It is particularly dramatic in people who have the *ApoE4* variant in both *ApoE* genes. More than 90% of these people are struck by Alzheimer's disease before they reach the age of seventy [60]. The ApoE protein has many functions. The ApoE4 form promotes the production of beta-amyloid peptides. [1]

Although genetic risk factors of Alzheimer's disease are known, it is still not entirely clear how the molecular events lead to cognitive degradation. Thus, it is possible that the plaques take up the beta-amyloid peptides to reduce the deleterious effects of the beta-amyloid oligomers. There are also inflammatory reactions in the brain, which can lead to attacks on the nerve cells.

ApoE also has functions that are independent of beta-amyloid. For one thing, ApoE supplies the nerve cells with cholesterol and fatty acids, which are important for nerve function; the ApoE4 form is less efficient than other forms of the ApoE gene. Interestingly, ApoE also plays an important role in blood vessel function.

Due to the prevalence of Alzheimer's, large-scale epidemiological studies have been carried out. (Epidemiologists investigate how diseases proliferate.) Only a few factors have a clear link with the onset of Alzheimer's disease. Particularly noteworthy is high blood pressure, which leads to increased Alzheimer's risk. A healthy blood circulation is apparently important not only for the prevention of heart attacks and strokes, but also for the prevention of senile dementia. An active lifestyle is, in fact, an important protective measure against Alzheimer's, as it is against so many age-associated diseases.

---

1 It is suspected that APOE4 enhances the function of gamma secretase and thus leads to increased production of beta-amyloid-42 peptide.

IV. Proteins, Molecules and Cells in Old Age

IV.1. Proteins: building, transporting, destroying

Proteins are like housekeepers serving the body's household. This chapter will explain what proteins and bead chains have in common, what tasks they perform, and why it is so difficult to fold them — especially at high temperatures, so that Quality Control needs the supervision of molecular chaperones. We will also watch how new proteins are sorted and dispatched in the post office, and how useless copies are placed in chains, adjusted and recycled.

The reason why a disease like Alzheimer's develops is apparently the accumulation of beta-amyloid peptides. Proteins, whether small beta amyloid peptides or huge proteins like the ones in our muscle fibers, must not only be produced but also dismantled or degraded. However, the degradation of beta-amyloid peptides fails in the nerve cells of Alzheimer's patients.

In recent years, the role of protein degradation in the aging process has become increasingly apparent. The machinery that is necessary for the correct construction and degradation of proteins in each cell works the way one pictures a highly complex construction site for a megacity. Buildings, from gazebos to industrial complexes, must be demolished if they are too old or no longer usable. New structures have to be raised. In the process, they are manufactured centrally, just like a state-of-the-art logistics company, and are marked so that they can be sorted and delivered to the right place.

In cells, just-in-time-manufacturing is a matter of course. There are two places where proteins are produced: the *cytoplasm*, that is, the "space" within the cell, and in a special structure called an *endoplasmic reticulum*. (Endoplasmic because this structure is "within the cytoplasm" and Latin *reticulum* because it looks like a small net or "reticle.") In the cytoplasm proteins are produced which are needed right there. In the endoplasmic reticulum, on the other hand, all the proteins are assembled that have to be taken to special sites within the cells, such as the organelles, the mitochondria, or the cell surface or membrane. All surface receptors are thus produced in the endoplasmic reticulum. All the growth factors that are released into the bloodstream have their origin in the endoplasmic reticulum.

In protein biosynthesis, the messenger RNAs (mRNAs) that we met before are translated into proteins. During translation, the sequence of the nucleotides in the mRNA is decoded into the sequence of the amino acids in the proteins. This process of translating mRNAs into proteins takes place on the *ribosomes*. The ribosomes are the molecular machines in which amino acids are linked to proteins. In the ribosomes the mRNA is bound and recognized by a special type of RNA molecules, the transport RNAs, or tRNAs. Each tRNA brings a certain amino acid to the ribosome so that it can be incorporated into the protein to be formed. By recognizing the sequence of the mRNA, the tRNA adds the right amino acid to the chain of amino acids, which results in exactly the protein defined by the mRNA sequence.

The synthesis of proteins is carefully controlled. The start of synthesis especially, i.e., before the first tRNA is loaded with the first amino acid to form the protein to which mRNA binds, must be precisely regulated.

Like any other biological process, exact control is critical. Nektarios Tavernarakis, Director of the Institute of Molecular Biology and Biotechnology, a globally respected research institute in his homeland of Crete, made an interesting discovery here. The Greek biologist studied nematodes that had a reduced amount of a factor that determines the start of the translation. In Tavernarakis' nematodes there was less translation and thus less protein biosynthesis [61]. Such nematodes lived considerably longer than normal roundworms. We will see how closely this observation fits into the concept of protein homeostasis, or short *proteostasis*, which describes the balance of proteins.

During translation, the proteins must not only be produced by linking amino acids, but also must be folded in the correct manner. In contrast to the DNA and RNA chains, which consist of four different nucleotides, which are all chemically relatively similar, proteins consist of sequences of twenty different amino acids, which can have very different chemical properties. Therefore, proteins are also capable of performing entirely different functions in the cell and in the whole body.

The pure sequence of the chains of amino acids is also referred to as the primary structure of the proteins. Then comes the secondary structure, in which a sequence of amino acids forms locally typical structures, such as a helical structure or a flat surface-like structure. It becomes more complex after that with the formation of the tertiary structure, which describes the three-dimensional spatial shape of the proteins.[1]

The shaping of the tertiary structure is extremely complicated, especially when a protein must find its way through the endoplasmic reticulum while sections of the protein are still being constructed that can greatly differ in their chemical properties.

The cell has various auxiliary mechanisms to help in the correct folding of proteins. If there are serious problems in protein folding, a quality control mechanism can be used, which can also lead to protein degradation. Incorrectly folded proteins can become a danger to the cell. They can really clump together. This happens, for example, if sticky parts of a protein that should be kept inside the protein structure are turned outwards and then get swept up with other proteins.

In order to avoid such unwanted contacts, proteins are accompanied by "molecular chaperones." In the late 1970s, Ron Laskey used the term "chaperones" for the folding assistants to protect proteins from keeping bad company; and proteins are always in bad company when they threaten to form aggregates with other proteins. Chaperones help the large, bulky proteins to fold correctly. Chaperones are activated especially in situations in which protein folding is particularly at risk.

The function of the chaperones has been investigated experimentally, especially after heat shock. Heat is particularly detrimental to the folding of the proteins. You can observe this in an extreme case when you boil an egg and the protein of the egg solidifies. The proteins spontaneously form aggregates and — as the chemist says — they "fall out" of solution. This means that the proteins can no longer move freely in the water but "precipitate" from the aqueous phase and form clumps.

In such an extreme case, proteins are entirely useless in their function; their spatial structure is completely altered. Under such conditions, of course, none of our human cells can survive. Human cells are perfectly adapted to our body temperature. Just a few degrees higher and we see the effects of fever. Even with relatively slight temperature increases, it is difficult for the proteins to adopt their perfectly balanced tertiary structure.

Therefore, the chaperones are activated as soon as the temperature in the cell rises. The chaperones can then support the correct folding of the

---

1 This structure can be measured using crystallographic procedures. In the late 1950s, Max Perutz and John Kendrew figured out the structure of a complex protein, hemoglobin. For this pioneering achievement, both received the Nobel Prize for Chemistry in 1962, the same year that Francis Crick, James Watson, and Maurice Wilkins were awarded the prize for elucidating the structure of DNA. A spectacular year in the history of the Nobel Prize!

proteins. In the endoplasmic reticulum, where the proteins are assembled, the *unfolded protein response* (UPR) reacts. These folding helpers are important for the cell to withstand possible stress situations.

Increased activity of the chaperones can in fact extend the life of the nematodes, but the importance of the various systems of cellular stress response is particularly evident in long-lived individuals. Thus, for example, nematodes whose lifetime is doubled due to mutations in the *daf-2* insulin-like receptor absolutely need the activity of molecular chaperones and the UPR. The activation of the stress responses also plays an important role, as we shall soon see, in an extremely fascinating phenomenon called hormesis. But let's keep an eye on our proteins as they move a little further toward their destiny.

Once in the endoplasmic reticulum, the proteins are already chained together in the correct sequence. Now, the folding takes place. The proteins are immediately labeled so that they can be sorted in the cell and delivered to the correct address. This happens on its way through the *Golgi apparatus*, a gigantic structure, which extends around the endoplasmic reticulum and is named after its discoverer, the Italian pathologist Camillo Golgi.

The Golgi apparatus is the sorting center of the cell and usually recognizes, on the basis of the first amino acids, where the protein has to go, whether it is in the mitochondria, the cell surface or other cell structures.

Proteins can also leave the cell completely, such as, typically, the growth factors or the structuring proteins that provide stability in the space between the cells. During their transport, many proteins are also broken down into smaller pieces. Frequently, small proteins, then called peptides, are extracted from giant precursor proteins. The precursor proteins often have the function of preserving the small peptides and then rapidly releasing them when needed. Such a thing is typical of factors that are needed quickly outside the cell when, for example, in immune defense it is necessary to react very quickly to invasion by a pathogen.

Proteins fulfill all the tasks our body needs. They are parts of molecular machines or have structural functions. They can be active as enzymes or as messengers and hormones. In humans there are about twenty to twenty-five thousand different proteins, which can be produced in slightly different forms in order to make up an estimated one hundred thousand different proteins.

In addition, there are various modifications that can be made to amino acids within a protein. Such modifications determine the properties and activities of proteins. Common types of protein modifications include the attachment of a phosphate group. A phosphate group consists of phosphorus, which is attached to an amino acid via an oxygen atom. For example, the p53 protein, already known to us, is only active when phosphate groups are added to it. On the other hand the transcription factor *daf-16*, which is so important for aging, cannot enter the cell nucleus after phosphate groups have been added and is therefore inactive.[1] By means of modifications like the attachment of a phosphate group, it is possible to precisely regulate when, where and how a protein is active or inactive. Signaling paths, starting from the recognition of a messenger by a receptor on the surface of the cell, are routed on the basis of just such modifications. The receptor begins with the attachment of phosphate groups to adjacent proteins, which then do the same with the downstream proteins and thus route the signal within the cell.

Like all structures, biological or man-made, proteins do not last forever. Like DNA, proteins also get damaged.[2] However, in contrast to the genetic information of the DNA, proteins can always be re-established from their gene sequence. In particular, proteins that are important in key functions, such as the regulation of cell division, are taken apart again as soon as they are made.

This is the case for the p53 protein. As discussed above, p53 activity has dramatic consequences: Cell division and cell growth are stopped — either temporarily or permanently — or the cell is driven into suicide mode, apoptosis. However, a functioning p53 protein is very important as the risk of cancer increases significantly when the p53 is missing or malfunctioning. Therefore, p53 must always be prepared to react to DNA damage in order to minimize cancer risk and render damaged cells harmless. But it must not be easy to get started and endanger the life and function of normal cells. Therefore, the p53 protein is produced constantly so that it can intervene when necessary. But the p53 protein is also most closely monitored.

It is the MDM2 protein that is responsible for this. MDM2 recognizes p53 and takes it to the cell's scrap heap. Here, MDM2 attaches a chain of *ubiquitin* to the p53 protein. The name ubiquitin comes from its universal ("ubiquitous") occurrence. With long chains of ubiquitin, proteins are marked to be moved to the cell's machinery for the degradation of proteins, so that they can be scrapped and broken down into their individual parts. The name of this protein depot, the *proteasome*, is derived from protease. Proteases are proteins that cut other proteins. The proteasome forms a

---

1 Only when the insulin-like *daf-2* receptor is less active does *daf-16* lose its phosphate groups, enters the cell nucleus and activate the transcription of genes that give the roundworm a particularly long life.

2 The big difference is, of course, that damage in the DNA can have dramatic consequences, because it involves irreplaceable genetic information. If the information encoded in the DNA sequence is lost, it cannot be recovered from anywhere. The DNA is the hard disk of the cell, with all its information. The protein can never be built right again once the sequence of the encoding gene is no longer correct.

structure that looks like a barrel or keg, complete with its many subparts. Proteins which are marked with a ubiquitin chain are placed into this barrel and are cut. At the end of this, the amino acids of the dismantled protein will be free to be used in the construction of new proteins. The Proteasome is thus the cell's recycling center.[1]

Once again genetic experiments were done with nematodes, which have shown that this recycling system of cells can prolong the life of the animal. Several factors responsible for the labeling of proteins by ubiquitin chains as well as the proteasome itself enabled the worm to overcome stress situations particularly well.

The importance of the correct folding and the breakdown of proteins can also be demonstrated in aging people. The "Gray Star" takes away the visual clarity of so many old people. The world can be seen only through a veil. Cataracts penetrate the eye and lead to clouding of the lens. The formation of these cataracts is a direct result of the aggregation, the clumping, of crystallin. Normally crystallin is a soluble protein. But when it is damaged, whether by UV radiation from the sun or by chemical attacks by oxygen radicals, the crystallin loses its tertiary structure. Then it requires chaperones in order to restore the correct folding. If this is not successful, the crystallin forms aggregates.

Throughout our lives, our eyes are exposed to the UV radiation of the sun. During our whole lives, harmful substances such as oxygen radicals, are produced during cell metabolism. Thus, the amount of damaged crystallin increases all the time. At the same time, protein folding is done less and less well. This is entirely in the spirit of evolutionary biology, because the protein folding helpers, such as the chaperones, were not selected by evolution to function in body cells indefinitely. Thus the crystallin aggregates inevitably obscure our vision, as we grow older.

IV.2. Stay hungry to live long: caloric restriction

Starvation is known to be fatal, but can also prolong life. The "Target of rapamycin" (or TOR, which means "gateway" in German) is indeed the gateway to long life for small animals. If the cell is starving, it begins to consume itself and to recycle parts that are not essential to survival. So-called caloric restriction can help the individual living longer, but it does not help ensure its species' survival, since reproduction gets compromised. The big question for us is whether that gateway to long life is also available for people.

---

1 But not all proteins are as short-lived as, for example, p53. Only recently has the life span of proteins been analyzed systematically, and that has led to the amazing conclusion that there are even proteins that are produced only once and then they remain faithful to the cells for their whole lives.

Molecules that are not able to form a viable tertiary structure despite the chaperones, or that are no longer functioning, whether due to damage from UV radiation, heat or chemical attacks, are hived off by the proteasome, the cell's recycling apparatus. However, the damage can also affect larger structures, even whole organelles, such as the mitochondria. They are much too large for the proteasome. Instead, such structures are destroyed by a process called autophagy (from the Greek *auto* "self" and *phagein* "devour") that was uncovered by the Japanese scientist Yoshinori Ohsumi in the 1990s. Through autophagy the cell eats its own components. The nematode, for example, turns to autophagy during periods of famine. The cells can survive the lack of food through autophagy, where they break down non-essential proteins and recycle their components for building vital structures. The self-consumption of cellular components is an important mechanism that can prolong life, especially under conditions of limited food intake. If the calorie content of the food is specifically reduced, then single-celled baker's yeast, nematodes, flies, even mice live longer.

Nematodes can even live for quite a while without any food at all.[1] However, the starving worms stop reproducing. Just like the extremely long-lived starvation or "dauer" larvae (*dauer* = German for "endurance" or "long-lived"), they delay reproduction until times when food will again become available. In adult animals, however, the starvation period has to occur just prior to reproduction, otherwise the longevity feature does not play out [62]. When deprived of food, the animal's germ line shrinks.[2] Only a few germline cells remain, and they cease being active. The worm can survive for months in an immature form, whereas its usual life span is just two to three weeks. If the worm is fed again, the germ line regenerates. Offspring are produced, and the worm lives a perfectly normal two- to three-week life until its natural death.

But the food does not have to be withdrawn completely; even a reduced food supply can extend the creature's life — albeit not so dramatically. It is now popularly assumed that less food also means fewer of the harmful chemical reactions that can be part of metabolism and therefore cells and tissues could preserve their youthful functions longer. But contrary to intuitive conceptions, the extended lifetime under limited food intake is an actively adjusted process.

---

1 A particularly impressive example of this is the dauer larval stage already mentioned. Dauer larvae can live up to ten times longer than a well-fed adult worm. But even adult worms can live without food very much longer than their well-fed siblings.

2 By the way, the same genes are necessary that encode programmed cell death in *C. elegans*. The precise function of the apoptosis genes in the reconstruction of the germ line in starving worms is currently unknown.

In the case of dauer larvae, we have already learned that the activity of the signaling pathway that originates from the *daf-2* receptor is critical. So far, the effects of hunger during adult life have been much less well understood — this life-extending effect was only discovered a few years ago. Longevity under reduced food intake is also determined by the *daf* genes. In addition, a number of genes have been discovered that regulate the metabolism and the stress responses with which the roundworm reacts to food shortages. An important role is played by a complex of proteins called the *target of rapamycin* (TOR). A lack of sugar in the diet, for example, reduces the activity of TOR, which leads to changes in metabolism and also to a reduction in the translation, i.e., the production of proteins. Let us remember Tavernarakis' discovery that reduced translation itself can prolong life, so that once again there is a clear overlap of mechanisms which determine the life span.

However, what is most interesting to note about TOR is that, as the name suggests (target of rapamycin), it has a pharmacologically active substance, rapamycin, that specifically targets TOR and inhibits its activity. Indeed, the simple addition of rapamycin can extend life. Is this equally true of mice and men? We'll get to that soon. Interestingly, when the dietary intake is reduced, the life span is regulated not only by means of certain genes but also by certain nerve cells' sensory perception of the environment.[1] If a lack of nutrients limits the amino acids available to a nematode, these nerve cells signal various tissues of the animal to go into starvation mode and ignite a host of stress responses. These include proteins that de-activate reactive oxygen species (ROS) and thus protect the cells from attack. In addition, the

---

1 Leonard Guarente, already known to us from his yeast studies with Sirtuins, concentrated on two distinct nerve cells which produce the transcription factor SKN-1 in the roundworm. SKN-1 plays an important role during normal development in the embryo. After embryonic development, SKN-1 is produced in two quite specific nerve cells, the ASI neurons. In these two nerve cells, under conditions of reduced food SKN-1 initiates a gene expression program that allows the worm to live for a very long time, similar to the DAF-16 transcription factor with low insulin activity. [63] The special feature of the SKN-1 function is that SKN-1 is only active in the two ASI nerve cells but still has effects on the entire organism. Such systemic effects are of particular importance for the aging process. In mice, we have already seen this in the hormonal regulation of body growth in combination with the longevity of Snell and Ames dwarf mice. In the dwarf mice, defects in the pituitary gland result in reduced body growth and prolonged life. But how can the organism perceive that the nutritional value of its food is about to be reduced? Interestingly, the effects of reduced food intake can be reversed by the addition of amino acids, components of proteins. In contrast to sugars and fats, which can be built (with only a few exceptions) by cells themselves, essential amino acids must be absorbed with the food. Thus, humans must absorb ten of the twenty amino acids from which all human proteins are built from the outside with the food; the other ten can be made by our cells. Chanhee Kang and Leon Avery from Dallas made an interesting discovery as to how a roundworm can sense the amino acids. They identified two receptors that sense a specific amino acid in a particular nerve cell [64].

proteasome and autophagy machineries are stimulated to release all reserves; it's as though the organism is just running on the back burner.

Not only in simple animal forms, but even in the case of mammals, life expectancy is increased by a reduction in the supply of food. As early as the 1930s, experiments with rats showed that reduced caloric intake can lead to a longer life. However, unlike with nematodes, in mammals the food supply cannot be cut off completely. Total starvation is just as deadly for rats and mice as it is for us humans. Mice also typically stop drinking when they are not eating — not a very healthy pattern of behavior. If the composition of the chow given to mice is changed so that the same volume of food contains fewer calories, the mice live longer. The assumption is that the production of proteins, i.e., the translation, is reduced as a result of the amino acid deficiency, just as it is in the nematode. And precisely that reduced build-up of proteins can reduce the protein folding stress and thus relieve the chaperones.

In mice, the life-prolonging calorie reduction can go up to forty percent; then they lose a dramatic percentage of body weight. Under such conditions of hunger, reproductive activity comes to a halt, in the worm as it does in the mouse. Their life is clearly prolonged at the cost of reproduction. Hungry animals are not in a position to produce offspring.

Dietary restriction with a specific reduction of the caloric content in the food provided, also called caloric restriction, has a life-prolonging effect in all the important model systems used worldwide to study the process of aging, namely baker's yeast, the nematode, the fruit fly and the mouse.

In all of these organisms, dietary reduction also leads to a reduction in reproduction. Even baker's yeast does not multiply in an environment that does not contain enough nutrients. The strategy is obvious, for how would a descendant grow to maturity without having food enough to be able to form all its new structures? A mature organism, on the other hand, has considerable reserves that can be recycled by means of the proteasome and autophagy. An embryo, on the other hand, is fully programmed for *anabolism*, the process by which living organisms construct molecules from simpler material, synthesizing more complex structures. It is quite possible that food reduction leads to the prolongation of life because resources are released which would otherwise be invested in procreation. In fact, animals such as nematodes, fruit flies and mice use a very significant portion of their energy to produce offspring.

The simple assumption that under conditions of reduced food supply the body can, at the expense of reproduction, extend its own life, has been questioned by the director of the Max Planck Institute for the Biology of Aging in Cologne, Linda Partridge [65]. Partridge selectively added proteins to the calorie-restricted diet of fruit fly embryos, and after that the caloric restriction no longer produced the effects of stopping reproduction and maximizing the life span. When she, however, only added the amino acid methionine to the calorie-restricted diet, the flies recovered their fertility — but they still lived longer. Partridge had thus proved that the prolongation of life does not necessarily require giving up fertility, procreation. Life extension could thus be achieved without sacrificing future offspring.

How would humans react to a drastic reduction in the caloric content of his food? Could a low calorie diet extend our lives? Prevent aging-related diseases? The results in simpler animal species suggest that caloric restriction may even lead to universal longevity. A contrary theoretical argument, however, is offered by the evolutionary biologist Thomas Kirkwood, who points out that primates such as monkeys and humans (in contrast to roundworms, flies and mice) expend only a relatively small part of their physical resources on reproduction. But how does caloric restriction affect primates? Conducting research on the life of primates is no trivial matter. Just like us humans, our close relatives also live a long life, especially in captivity. But an experiment with controlled food intake can only be carried out in captivity. Two long-term studies have been conducted on rhesus monkeys, with surprisingly different results.

The study by the National Primate Research Center at the Wisconsin University in Madison [66] was reported first. Ricki Colman and Richard Weindruch observed that a sustained thirty-percent reduction in caloric content reduces the occurrence of typical aging disorders such as diabetes, cancer and cardiovascular disease. In addition, the investigators noted that the gray matter was better preserved — an indicator that the nerve cells were better retained by the primates. The monkeys' life span was not generally changed over the course of the study. The authors of the study, however, paid particular attention to deaths that resulted from old age and found that the age-related mortality was reduced in the calorie-restricted primates.

A second team led by Julie Mattison, Donald Ingram and Rafael de Cabo launched a similar long-term experiment at the National Institute on Aging in Maryland. In this study there was no significant prolongation of life. The caloric restriction was quite sufficient to prevent any obesity but did not prevent cardiovascular diseases and some animals still became diabetic. However, in agreement with the Wisconsin study the monkeys in Maryland developed strikingly fewer tumors while on the calorie-restriction diet.

On the whole, when compared to tremendous longevity effects seen in simpler organisms, the results in terms of the benefits to life expectancy in primates were rather sobering despite some improvement on the animals' health. However, the reduced cancer development that was consistently seen in the primates as well as in earlier rodent studies raise hopes that reduced calorie intake could prevent cancer in humans.

Despite the uncertain effects on human life span, some people already today are placing great expectations in calorie-restriction regimens. Members of clubs such as the American "Calorie-Restriction Society" keep close track on their cholesterol levels and analyze each food ingredient precisely before consuming it. The jury is still out on whether these people are doing their health and longevity a great favor –but time will tell.

A variety of studies are presently being carried out to analyze the effects of caloric restriction in humans. There are positive effects, especially among people who suffer from obesity. Obesity has nowadays assumed pandemic proportions and has become a major disease of civilization. Particularly dramatic is the situation in children who are getting fat at a young age. While obesity was initially considered a US phenomenon, Europe has now also been caught by the fattening wave. But it is not only industrialized countries; even emerging and developing countries are being hit by the pandemic. Many children of the new middle and upper classes in China, traditionally a stronghold of slim people, suffer from obesity. In today's Mexico already the greater part of the population is overweight. It seems as if radical changes in eating habits are sufficient to cause pathological obesity. In the US, the problem especially affects Latin American immigrants. According to estimates, almost all Latinas in the USA are overweight.

In this context a study by the German metabolism researcher, Jens Brüning, is quite interesting. When he fed mice a high fat diet during lactation, he realized that their offspring developed irreversible damage in the development of specific neurons that control the feeling of satiety resulting in diabetes and obesity later in their lives [68]. The developmental stage during which young mice react so sensitively to the mother's diet would correspond to the third trimester of human pregnancy. It is therefore conceivable that an unhealthy diet is already transferred to the next generation in its earliest developmental stages. Caloric restriction may have little positive effects in normal-fed primates and probably also in non-overweight people. However, a healthier, balanced and reduced-calorie diet is urgently needed in the current obesity pandemic.

It is important to better understand the intricate biological mechanisms through which calorie restriction impacts on health and longevity. Even in the nematode, the genetic components of calorie restriction are not yet completely understood. The complexity of the composition of food should not be underestimated. It is therefore possible that people react quite differently to changes in the calorie content as well as the composition of their food. How different individuals may react became evident from studies with mice of different genetic makeup. Worldwide, scientists have used a handful of different mouse strains that have emerged from generations of inbreeding. Caloric restriction does not lead to life prolongation in all these different mouse strains and some even respond negatively. There are apparently genetic factors that determine whether hunger periods have positive health consequences.

An important goal of the research on calorie restriction is the development of pharmacological substances, which could be administered as a drug to exert the same positive effect in the body. De-activation of the TOR complex by means of rapamycin, for example, has the same effects as caloric restriction. Indeed, when rapamycin was administered in a large-scale study to different mouse strains in different laboratories, the animals' lifespan was consistently extended even when the drug was provided only from mid-age onwards [69].

Rapamycin is an approved drug. It is used under Pfizer's trade name Rapamune for postoperative treatment after kidney transplants. As was recognized by Peter Medawar, whom we've already discussed, foreign organs and tissues trigger the recipient's immune defense. Although they are life-saving for transplant patients, the cells of the transplanted organs appear to the immune system to be foreign invaders. Rapamycin can also act on the TOR complex in immune cells and thus reduce its activity. This is followed by a suppression of immune defense, immunosuppression, whereby the transplanted organ is no longer repelled. Immune suppression is essential after transplantation.

Patients must, of course, be well protected against infections. Under normal circumstances, immunosuppression is highly dangerous. Ultimately, our body is constantly exposed to infectious germs. There are even indications that caloric restriction could harm our immune defense. Possibly, this is a direct effect of reduced TOR activity under reduced food intake. The immune defense function did not play much of a role in any of the model systems in the previously discussed experiments on life prolongation through caloric restriction. The experimental animals were in clean, almost germ-free laboratories. How caloric restriction would affect them in their natural environment remains unexplored. Efforts are currently being made to identify more specific drugs in the hope of gaining the benefits of caloric restriction without having to accept the adverse effects of treatment with rapamycin. Alternatively, low dose rapamycin treatment, as currently pursued by Novartis researchers, appears not to harm the immune system and might potentially still harness some beneficial effects.

IV.3. Mitochondria: the power plants of the cell

Power plants produce energy but they also produce pollutants. It is no different in cells, which coincidentally create free radicals. The immune system uses these radicals as weapons, but they do collateral damage in the cell itself, which can lead to hearing loss, Parkinson's, Huntington's disease or organ damage.

The positive effects of caloric restriction are caused in part by *autophagy*, the process through which cells disassemble and recycle their own structures. When the cells consume their own constituent components, damaged structures of the cells are dismantled, while at the same time amino acids are provided that can be used in the construction of important new proteins. One particularly important target of autophagy is whole organelles within the cells. The dismantling of mitochondria is also called *mitophagy* because of its special significance.

Mitochondria are the cells' power plants. Cells process molecules such as glucose into carbon dioxide and water, a process called *cellular respiration* that takes place in the mitochondria, and as a by-product they generate a small but energy-rich molecule called *adenosine triphosphate*, ATP for short.[1] Cells can then use the ATP for any energy-consuming activities necessary. The German-American biochemist Fritz Lipmann, for whom the Leibniz Institute on Aging – Fritz Lipmann Institute (FLI) in Jena was named, recognized the function of ATP in transferring energy in intra-cellular metabolism. Together with Lipmann, Hans Krebs was awarded the Nobel Prize in the early 1950s for his discovery of the *citrate cycle*, also called "Krebs cycle." The citrate cycle is our most important energy supplier, in which electrons are provided inside the mitochondria, which are then introduced into the *respiratory chain*. Through the respiratory chain, electrons are transported along the membrane surrounding the mitochondria.[2] Since

---

1 ATP was discovered in the late 1920s by Lohmann, Fiske and Subbarow. ATP transmits energy by transferring its third phosphate group to other molecules and thus increasing their energy content.

2 The respiratory chain consists of proteins that carry electrons that are delivered from the citrate cycle along the membrane in the inner membrane of the mitochondria. During this electron transport, protons are transported through the inner membrane. The protons thus enter the space between the inner and outer membranes of the mitochondria. This results in an electrochemical gradient in which more protons are present within the membrane space than are inside the mitochondria, creating a potential in the membrane. In the early 1960s, Peter Mitchell published his *chemiosmotic hypothesis* — also known as Mitchell's hypothesis — according to which the high-energy ATP is produced by the membrane potential [70]. Mitchell was very isolated at the time; his hypothesis was completely rejected by his contemporaries. But Mitchell was found to be right and he received the Nobel Prize in the late 1970s. ATP formation takes place when protons from the membrane interspace are drawn by the *ATP pump* into the interior of the mitochondria, driven by the membrane potential. The energy of

electrons have a negative charge, they attract positively charged protons, which are pumped through the membrane whenever an electron passes by. This results in an unequal electric charge, because protons are continuously pumped out of the interior of the mitochondria. The unequal distribution of the charge releases energy, as we know from batteries. The energy is used to let the protons through a proton pump. It is precisely through these pumps that ATP is generated which can then be used as energy in the cell.

Oxygen is "inhaled" and at the end of the respiratory chain, electrons and protons are packed onto it. Oxygen + 2 protons and electrons = water. An estimated 98 to 99.9 percent of the electrons in the respiratory chain reach the end of this process and are turned into harmless water. However, some electrons react too early with oxygen and, instead of water, convert into dangerous reactive oxygen, a chemical radical, which can do all sorts of damage. When energy is produced, dangerous pollutants are always present, day in and day out, for a whole lifetime.

Reactive oxygen occurs in many different forms. By means of radical reactions, it can chemically alter molecules — whether proteins, fatty acids or nucleic acids such as DNA and RNA — and interfere with their function. In Harman's theory of aging, damage caused by free radicals plays a central role. Since free radicals are created in the form of reactive oxygen during respiration in the mitochondria, it follows that these power generators are given special attention in aging research.

For the cell, reactive oxygen poses a threat; it is countered by an abundance of substances and enzymes with which it can react and thus be rendered harmless. Although our cells have large quantities of these *antioxidants* to protect the body in an optimal way, a whole industry has been created to sell us other antioxidant products — vitamins, dietary supplements, pills and skin creams; But more on that later.

Harman's Free Radical Theory of Aging appears plausible at first blush: free radicals are invariably formed during metabolism, especially the respiratory chain, and have the potential to damage all the molecules of the cell. Because this theory explains the causes of aging so easily and simply, it has attracted widespread support. But even the most attractive and plausible theories have to be tested experimentally. After all, science does not simply paint pretty pictures; it has to identify how things really work in the world.

So how about the experimental test results on the free radical theory of aging? It is true that reactive oxygen interferes with the function of cells and, in the worst case, can cause the cell to die.

---

the membrane potential is thus converted by adding a further phosphate group to the adenosine diphosphate (ADP) thus forming ATP.

Our immune system also uses the deadly property of reactive oxygen as a weapon to defend against attacks by pathogens. Thus, when bacterial invaders such as salmonella attack our cells, they are fired upon with radicals and are destroyed. Not only bacteria, but viruses as well are attacked with reactive oxygen.

Thus it is obvious that the reactive oxygen from the respiratory chain attacks our bodies' own corporeal molecules. In proteins such attacks can leave traces in the form of a particular change to the amino acids. This change can be seen from the carbonyl content, a chemical change that occurs when reactive oxygen reacts with proteins. Reactive oxygen attacks on the genome cause many harmful changes to the bases of the DNA.[1] In flies, the carbonyl content of the proteins and the proportion of damaged bases in the DNA both increase with age. Flies that produce very high quantities of *superoxide dismutase*, SOD (an important enzyme that renders reactive oxygen harmless) actually live longer [71]. In contrast, the loss of SOD reduces the flies' life expectancy [72]. In nematodes, the results are less clear. The life span of worms that lack SOD genes is hardly affected [73].

Consequently, the importance of reactive oxygen as a defense may vary considerably in different animal species. Antioxidant enzymes, such as *superoxide dismutases*, *catalases* and *peroxidases*, convert the reactive oxygen to water through various intermediates, and make it harmless. If these enzymes were more active, how would that affect human aging?

To investigate this, mice have been produced over the last fifteen years to produce increased amounts of such antioxidant enzymes. The results were sobering, in general. In most cases, the life span of the mice was not extended [74]. However, Peter Rabinovitch was able to demonstrate that those mice that produce increased amounts of catalase specifically in the mitochondria do live about 20% longer [75]. Age-related changes in the heart tissue and the clouding of the eye-lenses, that is, the formation of cataracts, are also delayed in these mice.

What is the role of oxidative damage caused by reactive oxygen? Although the genetic information is encoded in the genome, which is protected in the nucleus of the cell, the mitochondria themselves have a small genome. A few genes are encoded there, whose products are used in these power plants of the cells. The genome of the mitochondria is in fact a relic of evolutionary history.[2] In the cell nucleus, the genes can be protected much better, for

---

1 The most characteristic form of such DNA damage is the 8-oxoguanines, which are formed when reactive oxygen reacts with the DNA building block guanine.
2 Today's mitochondria were originally independent bacteria. Remember the aforementioned *endosymbiosis theory*, according to which bacteria were taken up by the precursor of today's cells. But instead of being killed, as our cells usually do with bacterial intruders, these bacteria have survived. Their efficient metabolism

example, because the cell nucleus has the entire range of DNA repair mechanisms, some of which we have already talked about. The regulation of gene expression, that is, how much of a gene is read and translated into proteins, is controlled in the cell nucleus by much more precisely operating mechanisms than in the relatively simple mitochondria.[1] Mitochondria use simple versions of the machineries for gene regulation and for copying their small genome. And only a few DNA repair mechanisms are active in mitochondria. Nevertheless, in order to be functional, the DNA of the mitochondria is present in multiple copies in each individual mitochondrion, more or less in accordance with the principle of quantity, not quality. So if one DNA molecule is damaged, another one can be used.

Cell types that are particularly respiratory-active, such as muscle cells, have thousands of mitochondria. However, in recent years, improved imaging methods have shown that mitochondria are not usually present as single organelles but fuse to form elaborate networks with one another. If the cells are under stress, however, the mitochondria separate into individual organelles. The process of fusion and separation allows mitochondria to react to altered conditions of cell metabolism, for example under conditions of stress and nutritional deficiencies.

If mitochondria are damaged, they are "eaten" by their own autophagy. This process, mitophagy, dismantles them so their ingredients can be recycled in the cell. Disorders in mitochondrial dynamics or mitophagy can have drastic consequences especially for those cells that have a high energy demand.

Our nerve cells, or neurons, have a particularly active energy metabolism. The long extensions of neurons — called axons — transmit signals to other neurons or muscle fibers and thus pass on information. Just like cables passing on information through electric charges, axons are wires that can forward information through short and long distances. The axons can be extremely long, such as those of the motor nerve cells in the spinal cord that

---

suited the eukaryotic cells, which in contrast to bacteria store their genome in their cell nucleus, perfectly well. There was a mutual benefit for both organisms, so they entered into an inner symbiosis, or *endosymbiosis*. The bacteria co-exist peacefully with the eukaryotic cells, and they are not killed. Gradually, genes developed in the cell nucleus, whose products, the proteins, were brought into the mitochondria. Fewer and fewer genes had to be coded in the mitochondria themselves. Instead genes used for the mitochondria could also be more safely stored in the cell's nucleus.

1 The remaining genes in the mitochondrial genome are an example of remnants of times past, for nature, as we see it today, is only an interim product of evolution. We can see this very well when it comes to ourselves. Certainly, a human is a highly developed organism, especially when we imagine that in ancient times we originated from a single cell, from which worms, flies, and all other creatures were born as well. But the human species may develop even further. Perhaps a new species will emerge from the human being, some day in the distant future.

control the foot muscles with their extensions. Mitochondria are present not only in the cell body itself but also at the ends of the axons to provide the energy for signal transmission to other nerve or muscle cells. In order to be able to transport a mitochondrion through an axon and then also to generate energy, the division as well as the subsequent fusion process at the target site of the mitochondria has to function properly. If these processes are disrupted, malfunctions will occur, especially in the neurons. Hearing loss is a typical example of the effects of decreasing mitochondrial function. Defective mitophagy can also have severe consequences.

Parkinson's disease comes in a hereditary form and more commonly in a sporadic form. Hereditary Parkinson's disease can be caused by mutations in the genes *PINK1* and *Parkin*. PINK1 ensures the functional integrity of the mitochondria, the Parkin protein plays a significant role in the mitophagy, i.e., the dismantling and recycling of mitochondria. If either the *PINK1* or *Parkin* gene is not working, damaged mitochondria cannot be removed efficiently.

Ultimately, the effects of the hereditary form of Parkinson's are very similar to those of the sporadic form. In the sporadic form of Parkinson's disease, so-called Lewy bodies occur, named after the German neurologist Friedrich Lewy. Parkinson's disease is therefore also referred to as a form of *Lewy-body dementia*. An important breakthrough in the understanding of Parkinson's disease came at the end of the 1990s with the discovery that the Lewy bodies are formed from aggregation, that is, clumping, of the protein synuclein [76]. The sporadic form of Parkinson's disease is caused by the clumping of proteins, similar to the beta-amyloid clumping in Alzheimer's disease. And as in Alzheimer's disease, the dismantling process of a protein is also disturbed. In Parkinson's disease, the neurons mainly affected are *dopaminergic* neurons called according to their role in producing the messenger substance dopamine. Dopamine is important, among other things, for motor control, that is, control of movement. Therefore, Parkinson's patients gradually lose their motor skills. The controlled addition of precursors of dopamine, such as L-Dopa, can at least temporarily eliminate the motor disturbances. As an alternative to medication, a surgically implanted "brain pacemaker" can increase the activity of the remaining nerve cells. Several electrodes are introduced into the brain and they give an electrical *deep brain stimulation*. This treatment may be invaluable for the patients' quality of life — but even this treatment can only alleviate the symptoms of Parkinson's disease. No ultimate cure has yet been found.

Alzheimer's and Parkinson's are not the only diseases that appear to be caused by the formation of protein aggregates in nerve cells. Also, the breakdown of neurons in the brain of Huntington's disease patients is caused by agglomerations of the Huntington protein. This is due to a snowballing genetic change in the gene encoding Huntington's protein. Every time it goes through DNA replication, the sequence of the CAG nucleotides is repeated, and each CAG sequence is strung together over and over with each copy. CAG encodes the amino acid glutamine. The long sequences of CAG are then translated into long series of glutamines when the Huntington protein is generated. The Huntington protein is then produced with longer and longer stretches of glutamines. This makes Huntington's protein not only useless but also dangerous. Because of the altered structures, it forms aggregates or clumps, and these cannot be broken down by the proteasome. The large aggregates now hinder the function of the nerve cells, and neurons that do not work soon will die.

But why are neurons so severely affected when damaged proteins have difficulties being dismantled? This question has not yet been explained. The main distinction with our nerve cells is that they are all formed during our early development. They are differentiated early on and are not replaced.

Neurons form complex communication networks with each other; the *axons* emit signals and the *dendrites* receive signals. These networks create memory and reactions. Perceptions are submitted and processed, whether optical or acoustic signals or sensations of taste or smell, or how the temperature feels. The complexity of the human brain presents us with challenges that push the limits of scientific possibilities. The molecular mechanisms of how nerve impulses are transmitted are now well understood. The question of how muscles are controlled by the nerve cells or how molecules can stimulate the sense of smell has been thoroughly investigated. Large-scale research collaborations on both sides of the Atlantic are currently investigating the big unanswered questions, such as how human cognition works.

Precisely because each nerve cell is integrated into a complex network with other nerve cells, it cannot be replaced easily. How could a new nerve cell know what other nerve cells it needs to be connected to? In any event, the connections between the existing nerve cells are highly dynamic. Every new memory, every new impression we gain becomes a part of ourselves by means of neural plasticity, that is, the change in the connections between the nerve cells.

Nevertheless, the human brain has a very limited number of neural stem cells, that is, specialized stem cells, which can give birth to new nerve cells. However, these can only replace nerve cells to a very limited extent, such as those operating in the sense of smell. Presumably, this is also a remnant of history. In very primitive animals, such as the freshwater polyp *Hydra*, nerve cells are regenerated quite routinely. In the complex networks of the human brain, however, this is simply not feasible.

Nerve cells have an active metabolism and high demands for energy. Thus, they do not do well during an interruption of the blood supply, which carries the oxygen they need for energy production. This is precisely why strokes are so dangerous for humans — the nerve cells are very sensitive when the blood supply is cut off. A stroke can cause the death of nerve cells in very short order. It is so crucial that the blood supply be restored to the brain as quickly as possible. However, nerve cells are also sensitive to possible disturbances by proteins, which have accumulated to form aggregates. While other cell types in the body can be replaced, a malfunction or even the death of nerve cells in the brain generally is an irretrievable loss.

We already discovered how nuclear DNA damage contributes to the aging process during the discussion of premature aging syndromes. However, the DNA of the mitochondria, even if it encodes only a small number of genes, is much less protected. In fact, only a few of the repair mechanisms available in the cell nucleus are also active in mitochondria. The idea is widespread that the reactive oxygen generated in the respiratory chain attacks the genome of the mitochondria and causes damage. This, in turn, is a prediction of Harman's theory of free radicals, which are considered to promote the aging process. However, this aspect of the theory does not stand up to an experimental review either.

The modern possibility of determining the mitochondria's entire genome by reading the whole sequence of the nucleotides allows a precise analysis of the types of changes in the genome as mice age. Oxidative damage to the bases of the nucleotides of DNA leave a certain signature of mutations. However, such traces were absent in aging mice. On the contrary, mutations that occur during copying, replication, were found in the mitochondrial genome [77]. These mutations arise early in the development of the mouse when many mitochondria must be formed, so that many copies of the genomes of the mitochondria are produced. At the Karolinska Institute in Stockholm (Sweden), Aleksandra Trifunovic and Nils-Göran Larsson produced a mouse that makes a particularly large number of errors when copying the DNA in the mitochondria. This mouse ages in an accelerated way, just like mice with nuclear repair defects [78]. Damage to mitochondrial DNA can thus contribute to the aging process as well as damage to the genome that is stored in the cell nucleus. Larsson has even shown that mutations already present in the mitochondria in the mother animal can accelerate the aging process of the offspring [79]. Such a transfer to the offspring of mitochondrial DNA and with it the possible mutations happens in mice as in humans only via the mother; on the paternal side, no mitochondria are inherited. For only the nucleus of the sperm is involved in fertilizing the egg; the mitochondria are kept out.

If a mitochondrion is too badly damaged, it can be removed by means of mitophagy. However, if the compromised mitochondrion is not successfully destroyed, it can even lead to an increase in the number of defective mitochondria in a cell. In tissues like the heart muscle, where cells are not renewed by stem cells, such a proliferation of damaged mitochondria can impede the functioning of the whole organ.

IV.4. The life of grace of molecules

At this point we shall explain what life is, and above all what it is not: isolation. We'll look at why we need to understand how everything is connected if we are to understand the body and its diseases, and why we are in the midst of the greatest adventure people have ever seen.

But why does damage to special molecules, such as beta-amyloid protein, have such a drastic effect on our entire body?

Alzheimer's patients, including once powerful leaders such as Ronald Reagan and Margaret Thatcher, writers such as Nobel Prize laureate Gabriel Garcia Márquez, or scientists such as the physics Nobel Prize laureate Charles Kao, have lost their former mental power, while their memory and intellect were destroyed by a malfunction of a tiny protein. In addition, that's only one protein out of the tens of thousands that our cells possess. How can our lives depend so much on individual genes and proteins? All we are and all we think is destroyed by a malfunction that measures just a few nanometers in size.

Barely in the last hundred years, molecular biology has taught us that life is in fact a co-operation of the smallest molecules. But life is not simply the sum of its parts, as Aristotle already recognized. When the virologist Eckard Wimmer (mentioned in III. 3) published the poliovirus as a chemical formula, he made the distinction between a virus and actual living creatures. A poliovirus is $C332.652H492,388N98,245O131,196P7,501S2,340$, that is, a few hundred thousand carbon (C) and hydrogen atoms (H), about one hundred thousand nitrogen (N) and oxygen atoms (O), plus a few thousand phosphate (P) and sulfur atoms (S). A poliovirus is a quasi-living being, a chemical substance that can only infect a host, which then produces further polio particles.

A clear and everlasting definition of life will never be formulated, because of the diversity that distinguishes life on earth. Characteristic conditions, on the other hand, can be named very well. For instance, in order to be considered a form of life, a system must be able to maintain itself. A life form needs a metabolism, an equilibrium in an area circumscribed by the cell membrane. Life must be able to propagate itself, for example by copying the genetic material, followed by cell division. Life must be able to react to external influences and adapt to them. Signals must be emitted and received, such as signaling in cells by insulin or growth hormones.

But even a gene is not just a sequence of nucleotides in the DNA. A gene is a property. A gene becomes a biologically active substance only in the context of its environment. It requires signals that determine whether, when and how much of the gene is transcribed into mRNA. The mRNA can then be edited, i.e., various parts can be removed from the mRNA and joined to other parts. Thus, different forms of mRNAs are formed from one and the same gene, and thus generate differently formed proteins. The mRNA must then be translated into the sequence of amino acids to form a protein. As a finished protein, its activity can be influenced by chemical changes to amino acids. The stability of the protein is controlled by dismantling and recycling. All of these processes depend, in turn, on other genes in the cell, which themselves are also strictly controlled.

For this reason, a gene cannot be viewed as a single isolated entity. Instead, it is the interaction of the twenty- to twenty-five thousand different genes and the hundreds of thousands of different proteins resulting from them that makes life. Humanity has already taken a deep look at the functioning of its genes. However, we are still far from understanding the complex interactions of our genes in the context of our entire organism. Our brain is trying to understand itself; whether this project will ever be completed, we cannot foresee today. Our own self-discovery through scientific methodology, on the other hand, is probably the greatest adventure human beings have ever undertaken.

It is precisely because of the complexity of our body's biology that neither the aging process nor specific diseases such as Alzheimer's can be explained by the malfunction of individual molecules alone. On the contrary, the aggregation of proteins occurs in the context of biological interactions with other molecules of our cells and ultimately with the systems of our entire body. In recent years, a new understanding of biological interactions and causalities has emerged, in which they are viewed in the context of the whole organism. The discipline of systems biology seeks to derive its findings from the consideration of the whole system, such as the cell or even the organism. This approach is complementary to the classical inductive approach of molecular biology.

So, what are the consequences of molecular damage that make our bodies age and degenerate? For this we will now look at the effects of molecular damage on the human organism.

IV.5. The telomeres: protective caps of chromosomes and aging

Stories from the selfish cancer cell and the selfless body cell, which became a zombie cell! On the willingness of cancer cells to kill for their own immortality, the readiness of the body cells to die so as not to become like them — and about their fate, after death as a zombie cell, to continue to nourish the enemy. Telomerase as an herb against cell death — as the aging body leaves you in the lurch; and how we can change this — albeit with cancer as a risk and side-effect.

Of all conceivable damage that molecules can get, damage in the genome is particularly perfidious. The genome contains the information on the formation of all structures. Once the DNA information is lost, it cannot be recovered. That is why cells react so strongly to DNA damage. DNA damage checkpoints decide the fate of the cell. If the DNA can be repaired, cell division is only temporarily suspended. If the damage is too great, the cell adjusts its division activity forever and becomes a senescent cell or even commits cellular suicide, apoptosis. The damage is inevitably due to the inherent chemical instability of the DNA.[1] But damage also arises over time without any external influences. This has something to do with the nature of our chromosomes themselves.

As we have already mentioned in the previous chapter on DNA double strand breaks, strand breaks are an alarm signal for each cell. However, the chromosomes in our cells are linear instead of circular, such as the DNA of bacteria or mitochondria. The ends of our chromosomes are therefore, in principle, nothing but double-strand breaks. However, if they were recognized as such, the checkpoints would be activated in each cell. No cell would ever be able to divide but would be driven into cell death as long as its chromosome ends are seen merely as DNA ends, indistinguishable from breaks.

Therefore, the chromosome ends, also called *telomeres* — from Greek *telos* "end" and *meros* "part" — are well protected against detection by the DNA damage response. The telomeres are defined by a specific sequence of nucleotides in the DNA sequence. In humans, the chromosomes end up with

---

1 The development of DNA as a genetic substance already represents a great advance in evolutionary biology, compared to the RNA originally used as genetic material. DNA is more stable than RNA and less susceptible to small chemical change, such as a missing hydroxyl group. Currently, only RNA viruses still rely on this ancient form of genetic material; most organisms use RNA only for short-term functions, for example, to transfer genetic information in protein sequences by means of mRNA, to dock the right amino acid in the ribosome, during translation by tRNA, or for structuring ribosomes by means of rRNA. In addition, more types of RNA molecules have been found in recent years, and it is likely that *RNA biology* will still go on to provide some surprises in the years ahead.

long repeats of the nucleotide sequence TTAGGG. These bind to proteins, which prevent them being detected as a double strand break. Only as long as these proteins cover the ends of the chromosomes can they avoid the fate that attends double strand breaks.

If, however, the ends are shortened, the protective mechanisms fall away. A chromosome without protective telomeres signals to the cell that a chromosome is damaged. The DNA repair process then goes to work and can link unprotected ends of different chromosomes together. Such faulty connections of chromosomes can lead to instability in the genome or even to aneuploidy.

But every time the cells divide, the telomeres are shortened a bit. This is because the ends of the chromosomes are excluded from the DNA's normal copying process. The shortening of telomeres is not a problem for our normal body cells. Our body cells are not intended to live forever, as August Weismann already noted more than a century years ago.

The cellular aging observed by Leonard Hayflick in the early 1960s — his observation that after a certain number of divisions, human cells in culture enter cellular senescence, that is, a total resting state, and never divide again — happens precisely because the telomeres of the cells become shorter each time the cell divides. If the telomeres become too short, they are no longer protected but instead are treated like a normal double strand break. This is exactly when the checkpoints are called into action. The checkpoints then decide whether the cell should stop its division activity only temporarily, for example, to repair its DNA (in the case of short telomeres, a rather senseless challenge), or whether the cell should stop dividing once and for all, or even kill itself. Hayflick's cells did not enter into cell death, apoptosis, but into cellular senescence.[1]

Our body cells — never destined for eternal life — can live well with a manageable number of divisions determined by the length of their telomeres. The germline cells (sperm and egg cells) are, however, intended to live for infinity. Therefore, they cannot do without intact and protected chromosomes. A continuous shortening of the telomeres in germline cells would be the end of a species. Therefore germline cells use a very special protein: the telomerase.

---

1 The decision as to whether a cell with damaged DNA should kill itself or just stop dividing, by going into senescence, depends on the type of cell affected. For example, blood cells self-destruct and die due to apoptosis because they can be replaced easily through the division of stem cells or precursor cells. Hayflicks' cells were fibroblasts. Fibroblasts occur in connective tissue. In principle, they can be replaced, but even if they no longer divide, they can still give support to the connective tissue. Their dying would do more damage to the connective tissue than the presence of damaged cells that no longer divide.

The discovery of the enzyme telomerase must have been a very special Christmas present made to Elizabeth Blackburn by her doctoral student Carol Greider in California. The 23-year-old graduate student preferred lab work to festivities, and on Christmas Day of 1984 she had a breakthrough: In the unicellular ciliate of the genus *Tetrahymena*, she succeeded in detecting the enzyme that could copy the ends of the chromosomes and thus the telomeres [80]. For this discovery Greider and Blackburn were awarded the Nobel Prize for Medicine in 2009 together with molecular biologist Jack Szostak.

Telomerase is composed of a protein and an RNA molecule. Telomerase uses its own RNA as a template to produce a telomere-DNA — in humans it consists of sequences of the nucleotides TTAGGG. Telomerase is active not only in germline cells but also in stem cells, thus permitting the continuous production of new cells in tissues that are particularly dependent on renewal, such as blood or intestines. If telomerase is active, even body cells in culture can theoretically grow indefinitely. Since the telomeres are then extended again and again, no checkpoints are engaged to stop the division of the cells: the cells simply continue to grow. The attentive reader will not have overlooked the dangers of continual cell growth. Cancer cells turn on telomerase and thus secure their own immortality! Telomerase is therefore a double-edged sword. On the one hand, it is essential to maintain the regenerative potential of the stem cells and to ensure the renewal of tissues; on the other hand, telomerase supports the growth of cancer cells.

Carol Greider, now with her own laboratory (first at the Cold Spring Harbor Laboratory, then at John Hopkins University), and Ronald DePinho developed a mouse that completely lacked telomerase. To their surprise, these mice were completely normal. They grew normally, their tissues functioned just like mice having the normal telomerase, and they also lived just as long. However, when the mice lacking telomerase were mated for a few generations, their health deteriorated dramatically. Already by the third generation, the mice showed signs of aging before a year had passed, while in normal mice such signs are seen only after the second year of life. The situation worsened, and in the sixth generation mice without any telomerase activity showed dramatic signs of early aging.

People who have a genetic mutation in the RNA part of the telomerase or in *Dyskerin* (DKC1) — a protein that stabilizes the RNA part of the telomerase — suffer from growth disorders, malfunctions of the nervous system and a weakened immune system. The explanation as to why, unlike humans, the mice were affected only after their germline cells had ceased to maintain the ends of their telomeres over several generations is that the mice used by Greider and dePinho possessed extremely long telomeres. In these laboratory mice, therefore, it takes extremely long, even several generations, for the telomeres to be critically shortened.

The concept of telomere shortening was a much-respected explanation of cell aging following Blackburn's first studies. It was easy to imagine that the telomeric length could measure the age like an internal clock in the cells. The length of the telomeres does in fact decrease with age in the body cells.

Ronald DePinho did a spectacular experiment some years ago. When he switched the telomerase on again in mice that had lacked telomerase for generations, tissue degradation was reversed [81]. This experiment suggests that even existing tissue damage can still be eliminated. A hopeful view of possible anti-aging therapies! Similar results were recently achieved in another model of premature aging by Jan van Deursen, a Dutchman, at the Mayo Clinic in Minnesota. Van Deursen had deactivated the checkpoint gene *BubR1*, which is important for the normal distribution of chromosomes during cell division [82]. Without *BubR1*, aneuploidy occurs; the cells do not get the same set of chromosomes. This causes instability of the genome. The cells then activate the checkpoints and are driven into senescence, so their division is completely switched off. Without division of the stem cells, the tissues of these *BubR1* mice cannot be renewed and premature aging sets in.

A key factor that sends these cells into senescence is the p16 protein.[1] If p16 is absent, the senescence of the *BubR1*-deficient cells is prevented, and the mouse is spared from premature aging. Similarly to van Deursen's *BubR1* mice, animals lacking telomerase also benefit from the inactivation of the *p21* gene, which controls the senescence of cells similar to *p16* [83].

But van Deursen's next experiment was even more impressive. Now he developed a mouse in which the cells were killed as soon as they started to produce p16. These mice were also protected from premature aging [84]. So far, it had been assumed that the senescent cells, which never divide again, simply sit in the aging body without contributing anything positive or negative, but van Deursen's results revealed the harmful consequences of senescence. Apparently it served the body to get rid of senescent cells rather than to let them pull it into the spiral of aging. Currently, several labs are developing pharmacological substances, so-called senolytic drugs, that would selectively eliminate senescent cells in order to produce the beneficial effects that van Deursen observed in the mice.

Using pharmacological substances to deactivate senescence could indeed offer therapeutic opportunities for the treatment of diseases associated with aging. In particular, stem cells could benefit from abolishing senescence. It is conceivable that inhibitors of specific proteins such as p16 or p21 could improve the renewal of tissue. There is a risk associated with such therapies,

---

1 p16 is named for its molecular weight, 16 kilodaltons.

however, since senescence is still useful for our body. It is a natural means of preventing cancer.[1]

Already in the 1990s the American biotech company Geron was using the concept of activating telomerase to halt the aging process. This was a daring idea. Meanwhile, Geron has moved in the opposite direction and is currently testing substances that turn off telomerase to halt the growth of cancer cells. In principle this is a very promising approach. However, cancer cells are also known for their ability to conserve telomere structures in other ways, and the longest telomeres can be used by such cells to extend the shortest ones, independently of the telomerase enzyme.

Since the telomere length of our body cells decreases with every division, early attempts were made to estimate a person's life expectancy by determining the telomere length. In fact, the telomere length does have some predictive power. If a group of people are divided according to the length of the telomeres of their cells, the set with the longer telomeres does have a greater life expectancy compared to the other group, whose telomeres are already shorter at the same age [85].

However, the correlation, that is, the mathematically calculated relationship, between telomere length and life expectancy is relatively weak. Although it may be valid on average for larger groups of people, its predictive value for individuals is low. Nonetheless, Elizabeth Blackburn and the Spanish telomere biologist Maria Blasco offer commercial tests to determine the length of the telomeres. These tests are inaccurate and, of course, only give information about the telomeres in the cells tested, usually blood cells that are easily taken from subjects. However, the shortest end of a chromosome is obviously of much more importance than the average, since this is what triggers the checkpoints to take action when they read it as a double-strand break.

Telomeres therefore have an important protective function at the ends of the chromosomes. Since they are shortened with each cell division, the telomeres get shorter with age. The telomeres can be extended by the telomerase, which is active in germline cells and stem cells, albeit not in normal body cells. Telomerase is also activated in most cancer cells and allows them to become immortal and to go on with cell division until the whole organism dies of cancer. The "selfish" cancer cells thus accept the death of the body from which they have emerged, but ultimately they cause their own death through this "egoism." Our normal cells, however, are

---

1 In contrast to the positive health effects of switching off *p21* in mice that have been missing telomerase for generations, switching off *p53*, the key factor that induces *p21*, shortens the life of the animals even more. That's because without p53, the animals rapidly develop cancer and die quickly from the tumors rather than from premature aging [83].

"altruistic." If their telomeres reach the point where they are just too short, they themselves go into senescence and end their own capacity to divide. This prevents them from becoming "selfish" cancer cells themselves.[1]

Senescent cells have long been regarded as completely inactive scrap, which simply accumulates in the body over time. But in the last few years this assumption has turned out to be quite wrong. Rather, senescent cells develop their own activities and thus manifest a great influence on their environment.

The American Judith Campisi, now at the Buck Institute for Aging Research in Novato, California, has been investigating the behavior of senescent cells for many years [88]. She first observed that cells in the laboratory could be protected from senescence as long as they are kept under low oxygen conditions. In most body tissues, the oxygen content is less than three percent while it makes up twenty-one percent of the air. The oxygen must be absorbed in the hemoglobin of the red blood cells and then transported through the blood vessels into all the tissues. Particularly dense tissues such as those, for example, inside a tumor, may actually receive an extremely low oxygen supply. While cancer cells can adapt to this because of the flexibility of their genome, nerve cells in the brain are highly susceptible to reduced oxygen supply. If, however, cells are removed from skin samples or tissue tumors and further cultivated in the laboratory, they are exposed to an atmosphere with 21% oxygen content. That increases the formation of reactive oxygen, which in turn damages the DNA of the cells that are not adapted to such high oxygen concentrations. If the cell, in addition, experiences DNA damage in the form of double-strand breaks, resulting from attacks by ionizing radiation or chemical substances, for example, then division activity ends early and cellular senescence occurs sooner than normal.

The senescent cells do not die. Just as they do in the aging body, they can go on living in the laboratory dish for years. Their metabolism remains active. Senescent cells are particularly common in the vicinity of cancer cells. They could be inactivated cancer cells, which may have been driven

1 The regenerative capacity of the stem cells can also decrease if the telomeres become too short and the cells go into senescence. Moreover, senescence is not only a property of the aging body. Manuel Serrano and Bill Keyes, researchers in Spain, observed that senescent cells are formed in mice during their embryonic development [86], [87]. It is possible that the production of messengers from these senescent cells contributes to the growth of surrounding tissues. Interestingly, p21, the gene that drives cells into senescence during the embryonic development of mice, already plays a specific role in the roundworm to stop cell division; this allows the worm cells to be transformed or differentiated into specific cell types during development [88]. It is therefore conceivable that the genes that regulate cellular senescence in mammals, such as mice and humans, have been responsible for cell division during embryonic development since the early times of evolutionary history.

into cellular senescence due to DNA damage or after too many divisions. Alternatively, they could also be normal cells that were sent into senescence by the tumorous tissue.[1]

When Campisi administered an injection of cancer cells together with senescent cells into mice, tumors were formed far more often and grew faster than when cancer cells alone were inserted [89]. This gave her a hunch that the senescent cells released substances that support the growth of cancer cells. Campisi set herself the goal of identifying these substances in the coming years. To this end, Campisi kept senescent cells in their laboratory dishes for several weeks. Cells in culture must always be kept in serum; in the body, too, they are linked to the bloodstream, which feeds them with food such as sugars and amino acids as well as with growth factors — this is important not only for growth but also for survival. Without serum and growth factors even senescent cells, like any other cells, die. After a few weeks in culture, Campisi then took the serum to investigate whether the senescent cells had secreted any substances by themselves [90]. And in fact, the senescent cells produced so-called cytokines, small messengers that were known to be able to stimulate cells to grow or transmit alarm signals to the immune system. What effect do such cytokines released by senescent cells have on the body? Are senescent cells zombies, undead cells, devoid of any will of their own, that become the tool of cancer cells?

IV.6. Molecules are damaged, the body responds

Why DNA-damaged cells feed tumors, and how the immune system fights against them, often ending in comprehensive cell destruction. What this means for our aging process and the options for therapy.

Cancer cells need growth factors. We already know the Ames and Snell dwarf mice, which lack the growth hormone, or Kopchick's mice, which mature without a receptor to perceive growth hormone; they remain small

---

1 In order to study tumors in mice, there are three basic approaches. The more protracted method is to introduce into the mice mutations that activate oncogenes (such as MYC) or disable tumor suppressors (such as p53), and then wait until these mice spontaneously develop tumors. Alternatively the mice can be exposed to substances that damage the DNA and then trigger mutations, and then cancer will develop, just as it does in humans. These two methods take time but have the significant benefit that the resulting tumors are relatively similar to human tumors in their developmental history. If you just want to test therapies, often these procedures are too slow. In addition, the resulting tumors are often of different sizes and in different stages of development. Instead, it is also possible to isolate cells from already existing tumors and inject them into mice. This is usually done close to the skin. The growth of the tumor cells can then be monitored easily. When testing a therapy, it is easy to measure the success in shrinking the tumor mass.

but have a long life. Laron syndrome patients, who carry a mutation in the growth hormone receptor, remain small. We have met a whole mountain village in Ecuador, where a large number of Laron syndrome patients live. Both the various growth-impaired mice and the short-lived Laron patients are protected against cancer. Evidently, the mutations in cancer cells are not enough to keep a tumor growing, because cancer cells are also dependent on the body to supply growth factors. The young body produces these in abundance, so leukemia cells grow rapidly in children. In older humans, however, cancer cells often develop but the tumors generally grow more slowly. The growth factors are simply not there, because the aging body drastically reduces their production.

However, cancer cells themselves also produce cytokines, small messengers that control the growth and the differentiation of cells that tailors them to perform specialized functions. In addition, substances are produced which support the formation of blood vessels, among other things. Finally, a tumor also needs a steady supply of oxygen and nutrients.

At Cold Spring Harbor, cancer biologist Scott Lowe investigated the natural behavior of tumors in mice. He used a mouse in which he could switch on the p53 protein at will. We remember: p53 is inactivated in about half of all human cancers. Normally, p53 reacts to DNA damage and drives the cells into senescence, thus stopping any further cell division, or into programmed cell death, thus preventing damaged cells from growing into cancer cells. If p53 is missing, however, mice develop cancer just the way humans do.

The British cancer researcher Gerard Evan had already developed a mouse a few years before, in which he could activate the p53 protein in lymphomas, a form of blood cancer that had lost its natural p53 gene. The activation of p53 in the blood cancer cells did indeed have dramatic consequences: the cancer cells either committed suicide (apoptosis) or discontinued their division activity and became senescent. The lymphomas receded. While the mice without p53 died of their tumor burden, the mice with p53 could survive; up until the remaining cancer cells developed resistance to p53, and then the tumors grew again [91].

That is typical behavior for cancer cells: Due to the instability of their genome, they always find a way to develop new mutations. These mutations allow the cancer cells to change in such a way that they become resistant to any attacks, be it by chemotherapy or, as in Evan's mice, by the activation of natural tumor defense mechanisms such as p53.

This is done by means of natural selection, Darwinism at high speed. Most mutations either have no impact on cancer cells (for instance, the mutated genes may simply not be important for the cancer cells) or they have negative consequences, for example when genes that are necessary for the cells do not function due to a mutation. In rare cases, however, a mutation has a positive effect on cancer cells. For example, when a gene is switched off that is necessary for p53 to drive the cells into suicide or senescence. This was exactly what happened in Evan's mice.

Scarcely two years later, Scott Lowe developed a mouse with a somewhat different technique of p53 activation [92]. Lowe reactivated p53 in liver cancer cells. The liver cancer receded noticeably. However, the cancer cells did not go into cell death this time. Instead, p53 predominantly triggered senescence. Then Lowe made an interesting discovery: The now senescent cancer cells gave off cytokines, just like Campisi's senescent cells in culture. In the livers of the mice, the cytokines activated the innate immune system. Immune cells hunt the cells that release cytokines and then kill them. The cancer cells in Lowe's mice were destroyed by the immune system very efficiently. The liver cancer was completely knocked out. Immunotherapy, performed by the delivery of cytokines due to p53-driven senescence, is a highly efficient natural tumor defense mechanism of the body.

Lowe's research made it clear that cancer cells cannot be viewed in isolation. They live, grow and die in the body. They interact with other cell types and tissues. The immune system not only monitors the body for foreign invaders, such as viruses, bacteria and fungi, but also for dangerous cells of the own self. People whose immune system is suppressed have an increased risk of developing cancer.

This is a major problem for people who have undergone an organ transplant. Peter Medawar, whose reasoning on the theory of evolution of aging has already been of much interest to us, had shown in the 1940s that transplanted tissues are rejected when the immune system recognizes the cells as foreign. Therefore, after organ transplant, patients are treated with drugs such as rapamycin — which we had already learned about in terms of caloric restriction — because it reduces the activity of the immune system. For these patients, it is absolutely necessary to keep the immune system at bay after an organ transplant so that the organ is not rejected. However, this also has negative effects, including the increased risk of cancer. Immune defense against cancer is now a hotly pursued strategy in cancer therapy. This strategy has already achieved impressive results. In the future, it will be crucial to find a way to use the immune system to prevent cancer.

Cytokines that activate immune cells are emitted from senescent cells but also from cells that experience damage in their DNA. This is most noticeable in the skin after UV irradiation. We all know this: as soon as we've spent too long in the sun, the skin turns bright red. These are the consequences of the UV content of solar radiation. The UVB portion of sunlight in particular causes dangerous damage in the DNA. This DNA damage causes skin cancer.

However, the consequences of the DNA damage are not restricted to the skin cells alone. The damaged cells release cytokines into their environment. The cytokines in turn attract immune cells. In the skin the blood vessels expand, causing a redness of the skin. Heat develops as a result of increased blood flow. The immune system then contributes to the destruction of damaged skin cells; the discharge of cytokines triggers inflammatory reactions, which lead to cell destruction by activating the immune cells. However, immune defense has functions besides destruction. It also supports the transformation of the tissue so that new skin cells can replace the damaged ones.

The immune defense against the body's own cells can be quite militant. Its campaign against damaged cells can be crude. Often, too many cells are destroyed by the immune cells, rather than too few. The extensive destruction of cells also has its meaning. If, for example, the body's own cells are infected by viruses or bacteria, it often takes hours to eliminate the infection. Immune cells and pathogens are in a relentless race. Viruses and bacteria quickly jump to new cells and spread in the tissue. Therefore, the immune system attacks on a broad front. In the aging body, however, there is more DNA damage in the body cells. Driven by the leftover DNA damage and critically shortened telomeres at the ends of the chromosomes, more cells are rendered senescent. There is an increased secretion of cytokines. The immune system attacks again and again. This causes dangerous inflammatory reactions. Inflammation sparked by immune responses can also be observed in premature-aging mice. It happens when DNA repair does not work due to genetic defects. As we have already learned from prematurely aging children, the lack of DNA repair leads to DNA damage. There are serious inflammatory reactions in the various mouse models, such as in the mice that reproduce the Cockayne syndrome or in Hutchinson-Gilford progeria. These apparently result from the release of cytokines from the cells bearing DNA damage.

Thus the consequences of DNA damage are not restricted to the damaged cells. The damage has an impact in the entire body. The concept of systemic DNA damage responses describes this phenomenon that has only recently become known. The systemic consequences of DNA damage, which affect the whole body, probably play an underestimated role both in premature aging and in the natural aging caused by slowly accumulating DNA damage. The question, which now arises inevitably is whether the inflammatory reactions at the very least contribute to premature aging. In fact, inflammatory reactions can attack whole tissue structures.

In our studies of prematurely and normally normal mice, we indeed found evidence that the innate immune response was active in every tissue that we examined closely. In aging tissues, there is also such a concept as a "sterile infection," which describes an immune response without any bacterial infection being present. But what happens if the activity of the immune defense is stopped? Could this prevent attacks on the body's own tissues? Could this stop the loss of tissue function in old age, and even aging itself?

The human immune system is extremely complex. The most primitive forms of immune defenses are almost as old as life itself. As we have learned from Darwin, organisms are in constant competition, and only those who pass on their genes to descendants have evolutionary success. Many species are found today only as fossils. Think of dinosaurs, whose physical strength was not enough to keep them going. They could not adapt to changing environmental conditions. Genes must be put together in such a way that they program the organism well enough for the genes to be passed on to the next generation, because that is what it is all about. Every organism needs biomass, which it can use to build its own DNA, RNA and proteins. Plants can produce biomass from carbon dioxide and water because they have chloroplasts that can convert energy from light into photosynthesis. Animals do not have chloroplasts and therefore cannot produce biomass from inorganic substances. Even most bacteria need to use other organisms to acquire biomolecules. We know that viruses can only multiply while fully exploiting another organism, the hosts, whether bacteria or eukaryotic cells such as those in humans. So where does an organism get biomass? Of course, from other organisms. Eat and be eaten is the daily imperative in nature, including humans.

Most of the biomass that we absorb with our food goes into energy production (being warm-blooded, we need a finely controlled body temperature) or is excreted again. Only a small fraction is transferred to our own biomass for the building and maintenance of organs and tissues. The first forms of life had to be particularly good at getting biomass from other forms of life. A virus has to enter a cell and convert it into a virus production system. The virus uses the biomass of the host cell to make virus biomass. The nucleotides from the cell are assembled into viral DNA. Virus proteins are constructed from the cell's amino acids.

Bacteria pursue a similar strategy. In comparison to the cells of our body, bacteria are tiny. However, our body contains about ten times more bacteria than our own cells. Our own cells are therefore hopelessly outgunned by the bacteria in our body. Still, bacteria are very useful for us. They help our digestive system make food usable for our cells. Thus, a variety of bacteria live in our intestines. The advantage is reciprocal, because we feed the bacteria with each meal we eat. The composition of our intestinal flora is of great importance to our health. If our intestinal flora is disturbed, this can affect our health. In large-scale studies, it has also been shown that obesity is associated with a less versatile intestinal flora. The intestinal flora, also called *intestinal microbiota*, is sensitive to the type of food we eat. In the end, the bacteria are perfectly adapted to specific food ingredients. If we eat an unbalanced diet, the microbiota in the intestine can be permanently changed and lose its versatility. How, for example, caloric restriction might affect our microbiota is a very interesting question. But not all bacteria are well intended and help us digest our food.

Salmonella is not content with the food in our intestines but penetrates into our cells themselves. Then our immune system reacts and kills the infected cells. As a result of the massive immune attack on infected cells, dangerous diarrheal diseases occur. Stomach pain is often caused by *Helicobacter pylori*, a rod-shaped bacterium. This can lead to severe gastritis. *H. pylori* can even trigger stomach cancer. There is an interesting link between infection and cancer development. *H. pylori* can cause DNA damage in gastric cells [93]. It is therefore assumed that a permanent infection can lead to increased mutation rates in intestinal cells and thus to gastric cancer. Without a functioning immune system, we, like all species, are exposed to destruction. For five billion years, various forms of life have been in a constant struggle for survival. The real victors, of course, are the ones who pass their genes to the next generation.

But in every generation, a whole organism must be formed. Cells must be built for this purpose. Cells need organic substances in order to develop their structures. Every organism therefore needs to transfer as much biomass as possible from other organisms into its own. Viruses do this by attacking cells, bacteria by feeding off the food inside or outside of other cells. Fungi, for example, attack surfaces on the skin of humans or leaves and fruits of plants.

To survive this competition, you have to be able to successfully defend against other organisms. That is why defensive mechanisms were already developed with the first forms of life. Immune defenses can be quite simple in nature. A bacterium, for example, recognizes sequences of viral DNA and cuts them up and makes them harmless. Immune systems must always adapt to new attackers. The various forms of life have been undergoing constant challenges for billions of years. The attackers can shape-shift and escape detection by the immune system. Then the immune system has to adjust again.

Man has two different types of immune defense: the innate and the adaptive immunity. The innate immune system can in principle strike against any attacker as soon as it receives signals for the attack. These are, for example, the cytokines, which are also emitted by cells whose DNA is damaged or which are in senescence. The innate immune system consists of plasma proteins and cell types that fulfill various tasks in the detection of foreign bodies, the activation of immune cells and the destruction of potential pathogens.

The physical barriers of the body, such as our skin and mucous membranes, are also important mechanisms of protection from intruders. Most people know that a dry nose or a dry throat is sometimes sufficient to catch a cold. Influenza viruses then gain unrestricted access to our cells. Our skin protects a huge area, protecting the inside from loss of liquids and protecting outward from attacks by pathogens. A sunburn is a serious skin injury. Damaged skin cells die off, but before the skin can regenerate, the defense against external threats must be secured. The UV-damaged cells send out cytokines to call up the innate immune system. White blood cells such as macrophages show up, phagocytes of the immune system that literally eat up cells in the damaged tissue.

The immune response, however, must also be managed; if it spins out of control, further damage to the skin is likely. The immune system has also made provision for this. Regulatory T-cells flow to the site of the inflammation and curb the ravages of the innate immune cells. It is critical to balance between fast and effective immune defense and limiting the resulting inflammation. Excessive inflammatory reactions cause allergies when the immune system jumps into action even when there is no danger. The immune system can even turn against structures in its own body. Then we see *autoimmune diseases*, which can cause considerable damage to the body. In multiple sclerosis, the immune system turns against myelin. Myelin forms a sheath around the nerve processes and protects the transmission of nerve impulses just like the insulation of electric cables. If the myelin sheath is attacked, the transmission of nerve signals is disturbed.

The acquired or adaptive immune response operates much more precisely than the innate immune system. Evolutionarily, this is a modern and more complex type of immune defense. Molecular receptors on the surfaces of specialized white blood cells recognize the foreign structures of the pathogens. These receptors also serve as the white blood cells' eyes and ears. They recognize their own cells and leave them in peace. If their own cells are infected or damaged, they can be detected and eliminated by the immune system.

This property of the immune system is also important for eliminating prospective cancer cells. Immune therapy plays an important role in modern cancer therapy and is currently making great strides in the effective treatment of diseases that until recently had hardly any chance of a cure. The specific detection of danger by the acquired immune response is a particular challenge. The receptors must be constructed in such a way that they interact only with a very specific molecule of the aggressor. This flexibility in the construction of the receptors is achieved by mutations and recombination in the genes for the B- and T-cell receptors.

The immune response is not only highly complex, but it requires striking a very fine balance between the destruction of pests and contaminated or damaged cells and going too far, causing "collateral damage" such as in inflammatory reactions that can be severe.

The immune system becomes less efficient with age. This can be referred to as *immune senescence*: the reduced functional integrity of the immune defense associated with aging. However, the harmful effects of inflammatory reactions at the same time increase. These are presumably also consequences of the increasing DNA damage that has accumulated in the genome of the body cells over a lifetime.

How much is the innate immune system responsible for the damage done to body tissue in aging? The innate immune system can be switched off. However, a total loss of immune defense has stark consequences on the preservation of tissues. If such an experiment were to be done in normal aging mice, they would hardly reach the relevant age at all. Prematurely aging mice could provide some insights here.

Carlos López-Otín had been studying premature aging in Hutchinson-Gilford Progeria mice for some time in Oviedo, Spain. Let us recall that the envelope of the cell nuclei of the mice is unstable just like the cells of the Hutchinson-Gilford Progeria Syndrome (HGPS) patients. HGPS patients, and the equivalent mice, have stunted growth and age early. López-Otín was able to eliminate an important part of the innate immune response in these mice. As a result, the mice actually lived longer, and the tissues remained intact for longer [94]. Calling off the immune response, which the body was using in reaction to the instability of the genome in the HGPS mice, could therefore stop the animals' premature aging. Similar results were found in Pittsburgh by Laura Niedernhofer and Paul Robbins in another mouse model of premature aging [95].

Eliminating inflammation in aging tissues could therefore provide an important therapeutic approach. But the balance between successful defense against infections and the elimination of damaged cells on the one hand and, on the other hand, the avoidance of overwhelming attacks on still functioning tissues, makes it hard to come up with any simple answers at this point.

In the brains of Alzheimer's patients, the immune system also intervenes. For a long time it was thought that the immune system would be completely shut out from the central nervous system by the blood–brain barrier. However, the immune response is also apparent here. Microglia cells in the brain take on the job of destroying damaged cell structures. If a nerve cell dies, the microglia collect the cell remnants. Microglia also eliminate the aggregates, the clumps, of beta-amyloids, which are formed in the brains of Alzheimer's patients. The activation of microglia can achieve quite positive effects in mouse models of Alzheimer's. However, the immune response also has destructive consequences. It is possible that the degradation of the nervous system, neurodegeneration, has to do with the activation of the self-destruct function of the immune response. The immune defense has many facets. Simple switching on and off does not do justice to the various functions of the immune system.

Finally, the immune defense function is not limited solely to fighting infections and removing damaged cells. In recent years it has been recognized that the immune system also supports the repair and maintenance of tissues.

Only recently did we discover a completely new function of the ancestral immune system in nematodes in our research center in Cologne. The worm has no special immune cells, but only a precursor of our innate immune defense. It detects enemy invaders and then shoots them with antimicrobial peptides, small proteins that are directed against the invading microorganisms. In addition, the cells of the nematode send out signaling substances, just as our cells emit cytokines.

We observed that DNA damage in the germ line of the animal sets the immune system going in the whole nematode [96]. This immune response then triggers the body tissues to become highly resistant to various attacks from the outside, either through infection or by heat attacking the protein folding. Due to the increased endurance of the body, the animal is also able to prolong the time they are able to procreate, so it extends its *reproductive* life. Now we see a very clever response to damage in the germline. Essentially, the germinal cells are under arrest for as long as their DNA is damaged. Only when their DNA has been repaired can the germinal cells be used to produce progeny. This means the worm has to live longer, for the DNA in the germinal cells to be repaired and then new worms can be produced. From this we can see that even in the humble nematode, the immune system has developed features far beyond merely fighting infection. From individual cells, in this case germinal cells, the tiny messengers of the immune system swarm out to strengthen the body tissues' resistance.

In Drosophila, the fruit flies, the innate immune response takes over such systemic functions that affect the animal's whole body. At the Buck

Institute for Research on Aging in Novato, California, Heinrich Jasper focuses his research on the aging of stem cells in fruit flies. He has observed that flies stop growing when the DNA in their outer skin is damaged [97]. Jasper noted that immune factors were sent from the damaged cells, which in turn led to the reduction of insulin activity throughout the insect. As a consequence the growth of the whole body was reduced. This reminds us of the insulin-like growth factor (IGF-1) that controls the growth of the body in nematodes, fruit flies and mice.

The immune system also has an important function in regenerating the intestine in the fruit fly. This was discovered by Bruce Edgar, an American researcher working in Heidelberg, Germany [98]. The innate immune system also plays an important, though still little understood, role in the regeneration of the bowel and the skin in mammals.

Significant findings come from studies of the immune response in simple model systems. One important observation is that, due to messenger substances such as cytokines, local events can have systemic consequences throughout the whole body. In humans, these systemic effects are incomparably more complex. When it comes to hormones, it has long been known that they are produced locally but exert their effects in tissues far away. But the immune system can also produce effects over long distances. As a result of a sunburn, the local damage to the skin leads to weakening of the innate immune system in the entire body. This slowdown presumably prevents the immune response to the UV damage in the skin from over-reacting and causing too much damage in the tissue. Now, the most interesting question is how aging is controlled systemically.

IV.7. Aging and reproduction

The following chapter is devoted to the Methuselah effect. The center stage is taken by cats and mice that have played a significant role in elucidating it, as well as castrated opera singers and residents of mental institutions, eunuchs, the Korean Joseon Dynasty and the noble families Mok, Shin and Seo.

It is worth looking at simple model systems if you want to understand complex processes such as aging. Already when Klaas introduced his first long-lived nematodes in the 1980s, it was immediately suspected that they lived longer only because they invested more resources in their bodies than in reproduction. This argument was rebutted by Kenyon and Johnson in the early 1990s. However, the logic is clear, as the British evolutionary biologist Thomas Kirkwood explained in his theory of disposable soma (the body is expendable, once it has reproduced). The way the body allocates resources — to maintain bodily functions on the one hand and to enhance the chances of procreation on the other hand — is of crucial importance in maximizing Darwinian fitness.

Now, what happens if no descendants can be produced? What if no resources are invested in reproduction?

It was Cynthia Kenyon again, in San Francisco, who produced exactly the nematodes to test this idea. In the earliest larval stage of the worm, she destroyed two cells with a laser. These were the two cells from which all the germinal cells are formed during the larval development. Lacking these, the worms have no germ line. Such germ-free worms proved to be extremely robust and long-lived [99].

But it was not just the absence of the germ line itself that released resources that could be used to extend the life of the body tissues. Kenyon proved this with a decisive second experiment. In addition to the two cells that form the germline cells themselves, the young worm has two more cells, which are the origin of tissue for the protective sheath of the germline. When Kenyon destroyed these two cells as well, the positive effects that the germline destruction had provided for the worm's life span and resistance evaporated.

So the destruction of the germline cannot extend the animal's life if the directly surrounding tissues are no longer present. The key finding from these studies was that it is not just the allocation of resources between procreation and preservation of bodily functions but signals from the germline that control the life span of the body, even in primitive life forms like the nematode.

The germline also exerts an important influence on the life span in higher animals, perhaps even in human beings. It obviously has a very important influence on fitness. As we already know from the theory of evolution, the body merely serves to support the propagation of the genetic material through the germline. It follows that the life of the body has to adjust to the activity of the germline. The co-operation between the germline and the soma (i.e., all body tissues except the germline) is highly complex, like almost all the important processes in biology. That is why Cynthia Kenyon's experiments with destroyed germlines in the nematode were so important in recognizing that there are a number of active signals from the germline that influence the soma.

In mammals, too, removing the germline can prolong life, but not in both sexes. While male mice whose sex organs have been removed live longer, such a Methuselah effect does not occur in females. Even in cats, which as pets are often neutered, this benefits only the males. Neutered males live a good five, even more than eight years long, and thus about as long as their female counterparts when roaming outdoors. Indoor cats in contrast usually live a much longer live in any case.

Even if the removal of the female sex organs does not prolong life, the sex hormones still play an important role in determining the life span. This is shown in experiments in which the ovaries of mice were transplanted. Middle-aged female mice that had their ovaries replaced with those of young animals lived approximately sixty percent longer [100].

Does this link between the germline and life expectancy also exist in humans?

Here, we have to peer into the depths of the atrocities that humans have perpetrated upon their own kind, as castration has been practiced time and again in the history of humanity. This was done for a variety of reasons — in order to be able to hit the high notes as a singer, as in the case of the *castrati* of European opera houses, or to sterilize mentally disabled people (which was the practice until well into the twentieth century). In some state of the US this kind of forced sterilization of the mentally handicapped was practiced until the 1970s and occurred in some institutions even in more recent times. The Chinese emperors, Korean kings and Ottoman sultans were served for centuries by a staff of eunuchs.

As a rule the castrati lived just as short or long as their unaltered contemporaries. However, our life is difficult to compare to the artist's life, as they are usually not known for being preoccupied with health, either today or in earlier times. A systematic analysis of the life expectancy of neutered people was carried out in institutions housing mentally handicapped people toward the end of 1960s [101]. It turned out that they lived fourteen years longer.

At the court of the kings of the Joseon Dynasty, who ruled the Korean Peninsula from the end of the 14th to the beginning of the 20th century, eunuchs were kept as servants and guards. Boys would be castrated in order to be able to serve at Court. In contrast to their Chinese counterparts, the eunuchs of Joseon Dynasty were allowed to marry and to adopt children, and their adopted boys also had to be neutered.

At the beginning of the 19th century, Yoon-Muk Lee wrote the "Yan-Se-Gye-Bo," a genealogy of 385 eunuchs, of which 81 exact birth and death dates are known [102]. These eunuchs lived an average of seventy years and three of them made it to one hundred. Even the Korean kings died before they reached the age of fifty. It is exceptionally rare to live to the age of one hundred. The Japanese currently enjoy the highest life expectancy in the world, and even they have only had 3,500 people reach a hundred years. Thus, to have three centenarians out of 81 persons constitutes an extraordinary cluster of extreme longevity.

Now we come to the question of whether it was the loss of the male sex organs that gave the eunuchs such a long life. How can we compare their life spans to how long they would have lived, had they been spared castration? Since a direct comparison is impossible, a Korean research team studied the personal data of the Mok, Shin and Seo families. These noble families ran in the same social circles and led a lifestyle similar to that of the courtly eunuchs. The comparison was dramatic: The eunuchs lived fourteen to nineteen years longer than their unaltered peers. A man's aging is obviously driven by the sexual hormones.

That reproduction is closely linked with our life span makes sense, once one understands life in terms of Darwin's concept of fitness. Essentially, the body is there to ensure reproduction. It can only do this if the maintenance of its functions is optimally coordinated with the procreation of offspring. If the body ages too fast, it is unlikely to produce sufficient offspring. If it ages too slowly, it would have to waste valuable resources on self-preservation instead of using them to benefit the next generation.

In more complex animals, such as mammals, the successful transfer of genetic material to the offspring is not ensured simply by the conjugal act or even the birth of the young. Newborns have to survive a long time before they are, in turn, able to reproduce. In higher animals, the young are dependent on their parents, who protect and provide them with the skills to survive. However, the longevity of the parents is distributed unequally. Women live longer than men. This is true not only for humans; in most species, females live longer.

IV.8. Woman power: Women live longer than men

How seed beetles from Sweden and church records from Finland show that women live longer than men, and to what extent mitochondria, X chromosomes, and testosterone in this situation have a hand in the game.

Women live up to five years longer than men. This is evident in every afternoon subway ride. Even in retirement homes there is a sizeable surplus of the female gender. This inequality is no human anomaly: Most animal species show similar imbalances in life expectancy.

What accounts for women's longevity? There must be an evolutionary advantage; otherwise, aging would not be distributed so clearly to the benefit of the females in so many animal species. To investigate this difference, evolutionary biologist Alexei Maklakov at the University of Uppsala (Sweden) conducted a selection experiment with the seed beetle *Callosobruchus maculatus* [103]. He bred male and female seed beetles that had a particularly long life expectancy. While the females selected for longevity developed a higher degree of fitness (ability to pass on their genes), the fitness of the long-lived males decreased. These results suggest that ideally females still live longer, while males should die earlier to maximize fitness.

Is the longevity of women really an evolutionary advantage? Are women's genes selected to keep the female body alive longer?

Now, at first glance, the longevity of women is at odds with the theory of evolution. After menopause, women do not actively contribute to the preservation of the species. So why should biological selection still favor the further survival of the body after reproduction has ended?

This question was taken up by the Finnish zoologist Virpi Lummaa *of the* University of Sheffield in the United Kingdom. Her studies have caused quite a stir, again and again. Once Lummaa examined men over the age of 60 from 189 countries and came to the conclusion that those who were monogamous lived longer. Another time she examined the effects of birth-control pills on a woman's partner selection. Without the pill, women found alpha males attractive on the days when they were particularly fertile, probably because they promised healthy offspring; otherwise they preferred rather feminine types. But taking birth-control pills prevented these high-fertility days, with the result that women always prefer the softer types — which can have serious consequences for men.

To figure out why selection might favor the further survival of a woman's body even after she has passed the age of reproduction, so that women live longer than men, Lummaa studied church records in Finland. The church kept a precise account of which families had new generations to celebrate and when bereavement was lamented. Lummaa collected the data from two centuries. She analyzed how the life span correlated with the number of children over the generations, that is, how age is related to fitness. And Lummaa's team of researchers hit upon a very interesting discovery [104]: The older the grandmother was, the more grandchildren there were.

It was not the number of children each woman had that was the decisive factor, but how long she stayed around after she was past the age of childbearing. For each decade after her fiftieth year, two more grandchildren were produced. The presence of the grandmother was particularly beneficial between the grandchildren's second and fifteenth year of life.

Beyond his fiftieth year of life, the grandfather had no positive effect on the number of grandchildren. Although even in old age men are, in principle, still capable of procreation, at least in the historical records from Finland their role in procreation is hardly noticeable after the age of fifty. This may partly be due to the fact that Finnish society of the 18th and 19th centuries was very conservative and divorce was banned. Only widowers could re-marry and become fathers again later in life. However, such configurations came to pass very much at the expense of the children from the first marriage, who were less likely to succeed in forming families of their own. Consequently, male longevity failed to exert a positive effect on the number of grandchildren.

There is much speculation as to why men have had shorter lives. One valid aspect is that males compete to get a female. While the males compete, females face the challenge of choosing the right partner. And then, the mother's investment in the offspring is much greater, starting with the size of the oocytes compared to the sperm. While males theoretically can fertilize many females, the female has to be very vigilant about choosing a partner. In most species, as in humans, the male sex invests a significant effort to compete successfully for the favor of the female sex. Therefore, a full concentration of resources on early fitness is an advantage.

But there are also some molecular differences in the cells of each sex. The mitochondria — the power plants of the cell — are inherited only from the mother. The paternal mitochondria of the sperm do not penetrate the egg during fertilization. Thus, selection affects the genes of the mitochondria in the mother alone. It is therefore possible that the mitochondria are better adapted to the female sex than the male.

Another reason put forward for explaining the male survival disadvantage is that every female cell bears two X chromosomes, while males bear only the X chromosome of the mother. In each female cell, only the genes of one of the two X chromosomes are used, and the other is inactivated. In some cells, the paternal one is active and in others, it's the maternal one. In this way, the female body can better compensate for mutations in an X chromosome and gain an advantage. Hemophilia is caused by a genetic defect in the X chromosomes, and therefore it almost invariably affects men.

It has been said that the male sex hormone, testosterone, has a deleterious effect on the immune system. The only sure thing we can state is that men are selected for a shorter life. Apparently the male sex hormones play a crucial role in limiting the male life span. A better understanding of the effects of hormones and the immune system messengers is highly important for our understanding of the human aging process and for developing therapies to counteract aging-related illnesses.

V. The Environment of Aging

V.1. Lifestyle and life expectancy

In this chapter you will get acquainted with environmental pollution and with hereditary infectious diseases, and learn more about the modern, unnatural enemies of the human species: alcohol, sunburn, tobacco and our own nature.

In our modern society, life expectancy is higher than ever and is continuously going up. On average, our children will live longer than we do. Since our genes haven't changed much in the last two centuries, this suggests that other, external factors influence aging. What are the external influences that determine whether we have a long or short life?

Until the 20th century, infectious diseases were the scourge of humanity and decided on life and death. Prevention through vaccination and treatment by antibiotics has largely removed these causes of death. However in other parts of the world, infectious diseases such as HIV/AIDS, malaria, and tuberculosis are still the leading causes of death. It cannot be ruled out that due to global climate change, mosquitoes will again spread the malaria-inducing plasmodium in the United States and Europe. While nowadays malaria is only rarely seen in the southern tips of Europe, it was prominent in Antiquity when even warmer temperatures prevailed. Ancient Rome feared the disease that has long been known as swamp fever.

But communicable diseases are not the only health risks that have a dramatic impact on our life expectancy; there are many risks that we impose on ourselves. Excessive alcohol consumption in the long run causes liver cirrhosis; sun bathing causes skin cancer and accelerates the aging of the skin. A wide range of toxic substances can cause dangerous diseases, often through damage to our genetic material. Exhaust emissions in large cities can bring on respiratory diseases such as asthma.

The dramatic effects of air and water pollution are now increasingly evident, for example in China, which is expanding industrially. We already hear of "cancer villages" where inhabitants are reported to be victims of a ruthless level of industrial pollution. One short visit to Beijing is enough to show the extent of the acrid air pollution and to get a sense of the health implications, when the thick smog only allows us to guess at the vastness of Tiananmen Square and the Forbidden City can only be seen through a veil.

Smoking is the number one self-inflicted health problem. Both active and passive smokers breathe substances that damage the genome. Smoking not only increases the risk of lung cancer but also makes us more susceptible to other types of cancer. In addition, the toxic substances in cigarette smoke accelerate the aging of many tissues. We should not let the famous story of the "ninety-year-old chain-smoking grandfather" mislead us: The genetic constitution that makes the body react to harmful substances is very diverse and, so far, unpredictable. There is no doubt that smoking is an addictive disease that has a dangerous impact on cancer risk and aging.

V.2. Nutrition and Aging

Less is more — in the following, we learn a little more about the dangers of excess and the advantages of shortages, and how our society both makes it possible to live longer and at the same time prevents it.

Can a healthy diet or a certain regimen prolong life? In general, people believe that healthy food and a strong physical constitution protect us against disease and ensure a long life. Vitamins are touted for their promises of good health. But is there scientific evidence for such claims? Do we actually know exactly what is healthy? And is the same thing healthy for every human being?

The truth is that "proper nutrition" is complicated. We have already learned about caloric restriction. It was first discovered in rats, in the 1930s, and today hardly a species has been found that does not benefit from a limit of the calorie content of its food. Whether we are talking about baker's yeast, nematodes, fruit flies or mice and rats, they all live longer if their food intake is reduced, partially or even drastically.

The link between the longevity genes and the physiology of starvation is interesting. The long-lasting *dauer* stage of the nematode comes about due to hunger during the larval stage. The same genes that control the dauer stage also determine the life span of the adult animal. The dauer stage allows the nematode larvae to go without food for a long period of time so that it can survive until food is available again. Food deprivation also leads to a prolongation of life in adult worms.

For mice and rats, all we need to do is reduce the protein content of their food and they will live longer. But even in mice, it is not clear what is the mechanism by which calorie reduction leads to a longer life. Different mouse strains respond very differently to caloric restriction.

The situation is even more complicated in non-human primates. Studies were conducted using rhesus monkeys over a period of thirty years and they involved a considerable effort. As mentioned in the chapter discussing calorie restriction such studies have been done in the United States, one in Wisconsin, the second in Maryland. While the Wisconsin study concluded that calorie restriction could prevent age-related illnesses and extend the healthy life span [66], the study at the National Institute on Aging found little evidence of life span promoting effects due to caloric restriction [67]. The authors chose different compositions of food in the two studies. This alone shows that it will not be easy to apply even what we learn with monkeys to humans. We are also warned that calorie restriction could weaken the immune system.

One should bear in mind three aspects when looking at caloric restriction, before starting to experiment on oneself (as some people are already doing, especially in the USA) by strictly limiting food intake. First of all, the means by which we absorb our food is very complex. We do not ingest our food directly, but let it be processed by the microbiota in our intestine (gut flora). In human intestines, there are about 100 trillion bacteria — that's ten times more than all the cells in the human body. These bacteria keep the immune system busy; it has to distinguish between good and harmful bacteria. There is a correlation between a diverse microbiota and better health in older people. Up to one thousand different bacterial species can inhabit the human intestine. You need to have a diverse diet in order to have a diverse microbiota. The complexity of the intestinal microbiota, and intestinal health, are far from well understood. But it plays an important role when we want to influence our health through our diet.

The second aspect is how each species adapts to the food sources that have been used for millions of years. Humans have greatly expanded their diet. Until agriculture was invented over ten thousand years ago in Mesopotamia, the land between the Euphrates and Tigris rivers (today's Iraq and the north-east part of today's Syria), humans were dependent on gathering berries and hunting game. Farming apparently did not turn out to be entirely beneficial for humans. It can be concluded from skeletal findings that the human's body size has actually decreased as a result of the changes in food habits. Today, we are experiencing a paradoxical trend towards one-sided nutrition. This trend is driven by an industry based on the profitability of monocultures. A high fat content and a lot of salt also stimulate the taste buds. The taste of industrial food is enhanced by additives such as glutamate. Our taste buds adapt to this over time. We like the food we are accustomed to. It is not easy to convert to a balanced and healthy diet.

Third, nutritional trials are carried out under protected laboratory conditions. The mice used in experiments live in a clean and protected environment. Their life is not threatened by any infections. It is hard to predict whether their immune system would stand up to natural conditions. If caloric restriction weakens the immune system, for example, this would have little effect in the laboratory, but it could be fatal in the wild.

Thus, each animal species, including the human being, is adapted to a particular, natural food composition. This looks quite different in rodents than in monkeys or even humans. Therefore, caution should be exercised when trying to translate such complex processes as the effects of food on metabolism from a few simple animal species to humans. What is clear, however, is that the increasing obesity of our population, with more overweight people than ever before in the history of humankind, entails considerable health risks. A reduction in food intake will, of course, be health-promoting, especially for overweight people.

It is really an irony of fate that modern man is handling so poorly the rich food supply available today. Until the 19th century, Europeans were plagued by famine. Meat was a rare luxury for many people. Modern agriculture is able to produce food in great abundance, even though abundance may not be synonymous with quality. But there is an adequate and varied range of food available to every human being. But try to put together a shopping cart of healthy food in an American supermarket. If you succeed, it will only be at prices that are horrendous compared to cheap finished goods. A healthy diet requires effort. Restaurants are one thing — go to any of the fast food chains — you get fed in no time and the prices are so low that it is very tempting to stop in. It's easier to pick up convenience food instead of shopping and cooking fresh. Having a healthy diet requires a certain commitment, both in the selection of ingredients and in the preparation.

But it is not the food alone that matters. While our ancestors still had to travel long distances every day to find something to eat, or expend a lot of physical effort, we often spend most of the day just sitting. *Homo sapiens* led a physically active lifestyle for 199,900 years of its 200,000-year history. The urge to physical inactivity, which makes us sink into our TV chairs and comfortable car seats, is probably due to the resting phases that were necessary in the difficult lives our ancestors led. Physical activity is often preached, but few people manage to lead a consistently balanced lifestyle.

We have to acknowledge that it takes an effort to be physically active. Our needs, from the desire for food or drink, restlessness or laziness, sex or alcohol, are all controlled by our brain. Even though we might be firmly convinced that our behavior stems from our free will, brain research has revealed how dependent we are on the activity of our nerve cells. Although we still do not understand very much what human consciousness is and how decisions of the mind are made in the brain, our deepest instincts most certainly still influence our behavior. Making a rational decision after carefully weighing the pros and cons is difficult for us; it is just not in our nature.

Instead of deciding for the most rationale course, it is often easier to follow the leaders and idols, because it's instinctive and a highly successful survival strategy in social animals. Of course, this can lead straight to perdition. Like lemmings that plunge into the canyons, people have followed leaders again and again to mass death. But the social order of leaders and followers was also crowned with great successes in the history of humankind. It was just this power of social organization that led to agriculture and livestock breeding instead of hunting and gathering, which paved the way to civilization — despite the deteriorating food. Work could be distributed efficiently, and attacks on rival groups could be organized much better than before.

Scientific progress has, in the meantime, brought about an epochal shift in knowledge of ourselves and the consequences of our actions. Nevertheless, we have also remained animals. Making rational decisions is hard for us. We know about climate change, but we argue about what caused it. It's as though a tidal wave were coming and we wondered who might have caused it, instead of building a dam.

The same applies to our behavior toward ourselves, especially to our eating habits and our lack of exercise. It can be very difficult for people to change their habits. We therefore rely on convenient ways to eat healthier. What would be more obvious than putting healthy additives into industrial food? The industry is always talking about certain food additives with anti-aging qualities. Antioxidants in particular are praised, that is, substances which — figuratively speaking — are supposed to protect our molecules from rusting. Antioxidants have been used in many foods for decades to give them a longer shelf life. Antioxidants, for example, keep butter from getting discolored at the edges, so it looks fresh longer.

The efficacy of antioxidants fits perfectly into Harman's theory that reactive oxygen causes the destruction of cells. However, scientific evidence that oxidative damage plays a role in aging is anything but clear, as we have seen — but even more unexpected discoveries were to come. When metabolism researcher Michael Ristow fed his extremely long-lived nematodes, the ones with the *daf-2* mutation, with an antioxidant, suddenly the Methuselah effect evaporated. As young adults, *daf-2* mutants produce a blast of reactive oxygen and this temporary occurrence of reactive oxygen is absolutely necessary for the *daf-2* worms to reach a long life. Ristow's experiments showed that reactive oxygen, known for its harmful effects on everything that comes its way, can also have a positive effect on the life span.

Already in the 1880s Hugo Schulz and Rudolf Arendt postulated, based on their experiments with yeasts, the Arndt-Schulz rule stipulating that small amounts of toxins can have positive effects, while the same poison in high quantities leads to death. This phenomenon is called *Hormesis* — and it has been experiencing a renaissance in aging research in the past two decades.

V.3. When poison does us good: Hormesis

"What doesn't kill me makes me stronger" — How can we apply this bit of Nietzschean wisdom to our body and its aging process?

Hormesis (from Greek "fast movement"), is encapsulated in Nietzsche's oft-quoted saying, "What doesn't kill me only makes me stronger" (*Twilight of the Idols, Maxims and Arrows*). The term Hormesis was coined by Chester Southam and John Ehrlich in the 1940s when they found that small amounts of a toxin from a worm extract stimulated the growth of fungi while in higher quantities the same substance slowed growth [106].

Soon after this discovery, however, Hormesis fell under the long shadows of homeopathy, which is based on such extreme dilutions of substances that they are barely present at all. In addition, Hormesis is of limited use in clinical applications. It is difficult to estimate the proper concentration to use in humans.

For a long time it was not known how Hormesis worked. In recent years, gerontology research has spelled it out in detail. Edward Caprese meticulously combed through the scientific literature on Hormesis for about twenty years and he assigns a positive effect to almost all toxins when applied at a sufficiently low concentration [107]. Roundworms that are exposed to a temporary heat shock live just as long as those who have lived through periods of starvation. The heat stress and the hunger send a signal to the nerve cells, which then instruct the entire body of the animal to adopt a high-endurance state. This leads to the production of chaperones that help to fold the proteins, and the activation of autophagy, so that parts of the cell can be eaten up and recycled into the proteins that are needed the most. As a result, the proteins are folded more optimally and they are less likely to form clumps; the resources of the cells can be better utilized.

Stress resistance, i.e., resistance to harmful influences, is a universal property of mutants whose life is extended. This applies to the extremely stress-resistant *daf-2* mutants as well as to the roundworms whose germline was destroyed. Long-lived mice that produce less of the IGF-1 receptor (equivalent to the *daf-2* receptor) also show increased resistance to oxidative damage.

Can stress increase the endurance and longevity of tissues? Jay Mitchell and Ron de Bruin used mice as an experimental system for surgical procedures at the Erasmus Medical Center in Rotterdam (Netherlands). During kidney transplants, the blood supply must be interrupted. This leads to a lack of oxygen. When the blood supply is restored after a brief interruption, *reperfusion* (or re-oxygenation) injury can occur. The sharp increase of oxygen causes oxidative damage. Reperfusion has been shown to cause the same tissue damage in patients as it does in the experimental mouse system. Surprisingly, Mitchell and de Bruin observed that mice suffering from Cockayne syndrome [108] survived reperfusion a lot better. Don't forget, Cockayne syndrome is caused by malfunctions in DNA repair and leads to stunted growth and premature aging. These mice, however, also show less of the insulin-like messenger IGF-1, just like the long-lived dwarf mice, so clearly the organism responds to DNA damage by activating its longevity program and the associated stress resistance.

The next step, obviously, was to test whether caloric restriction would also make the mice impervious to oxidative damage after the blood supply is restored. Already after just a few days of reduced food intake, prior to surgery, Mitchell's and de Bruin's starving mice survived reperfusion much better.

Clinical trials are currently underway to test whether patients recover faster from kidney transplants if their caloric intake is limited beforehand. If successful, this would be a very simple preventative procedure with broad application in everyday clinical practice. In addition, meticulous research is being carried out to identify therapeutic substances that could offer the same protective effect as caloric restriction. Hormesis is quite evident in nature. Whether in single-cell baker's yeasts, the simplest multicellular organisms such as roundworms, insects such as flies, or mice, hormetic stress has a positive effect on the cells' resistance and the longevity of the organism. Can minor stress also promote health in humans? Whenever we play sports, we are actually doing nothing but subjecting our bodies to "stress."

In order to test whether Hormesis plays a role in the health-promoting effects of physical training, Michael Ristow studied the impact of sportive activity on two different types of subjects: a group of well-trained students of sport, and a rather less athletic group, to see whether sports led to any particular health benefits [109]. The latter subjects were recruited from medical students.

When muscles are active, their power plants, the mitochondria, are breathing. The number of mitochondria in the muscle cells increases continuously with regular training. However, the mitochondrial activity also leads to the release of reactive oxygen. When Ristow gave the sports and medical students a combination of the antioxidant vitamins C and vitamin E during their training sessions, the training did not show positive effects.

As an immediate success of athletic training, insulin sensitivity goes up. Insulin flows from the islet cells in the pancreas to activate the insulin receptor. This receptor sits on the surface of the cells in various body tissues, including the muscle and liver and fat cells, and sends a signal to these cells as soon as the messenger substance insulin binds to it. The insulin receptor then stimulates the intake of sugar from the blood and supplies the cells with energy.

The more sensitive the body is to insulin, the better the sugar is absorbed from the blood and the better the cells are supplied with "fuel" sugar. With increasing age, insulin sensitivity decreases. Overweight people in particular are at high risk of becoming insulin resistant, and then they can suffer from type 2 diabetes, *diabetes mellitus*. In such cases the insulin receptor is no longer effectively activated, and the sugar can no longer be absorbed into the cells from the blood. Not only does athletic exercise counteract the tendency to be overweight, it also reduces the risk of diabetes. During exercise, the subjects who did not receive antioxidants showed increased insulin sensitivity, suggesting that athletic activity did, indeed, reduce their risk of diabetes. In subjects who were given vitamins C and E, however, the insulin sensitivity decreased. Apparently, the production of reactive oxygen is necessary for the stress to produce the positive effects of hormesis.

What we have learned from the simple models also applies to humans: A small amount of stress has a positive effect on health. Initiating hormesis can improve the body's stress resistance and health.

The example of vitamin therapy teaches us another important lesson: Vitamins are undeniably important parts of our diet, which should in no case be dispensed with. However, the assumption that vitamins have only positive effects is misleading. Even much advertised vitamins like vitamin C could also have negative effects. Food supplements, such as vitamin products, should not be taken indiscriminately. Even if a whole industry is pushing vitamin products and they are freely available for purchase, this does not mean that they are good for you.

Controlled scientific studies are needed to assess the impact of food supplements. Antioxidants are heavily advertised, but their long-term impact on our body is, as yet, poorly understood. The theory that reactive oxygen causes molecular damage in the cell is easy to understand and is a simple explanation of what causes aging — but that does not mean that it is true.

V.4. Superficial treatments for superficial aging: Anti-aging cosmetics

But not only can poison do us good — what's good can also be poison! Here's what soap, the sun, cosmetics and the industry of youthfulness have in common with Silvio Berlusconi, Nicolas Cage and Jürgen Klopp.

Anti-aging labels are found these days on dozens of cosmetics. If new product lines like "CoQ10," "DNAge," and "DNA protect" all promise to rejuvenate our image, it's because we feel our age mostly because of how we look.

We usually only become aware of how old our heart is when we have a heart attack, our liver only when our blood tests come back with shocking numbers, our brain when acquaintances and relatives are stunned by our first signs of forgetfulness, and our bones only if a minor fall causes severe fractures. But men know when they are losing hair and women know when the first gray strands call for some good hair color. Wrinkles start to mask our features and old age spots dot our hands and face (due to *senile lentigo* or lipofuscin, a pigment that accumulates even in aging roundworms).

We place a special value on our youthful appearance. Our deepest instincts react to the outward appearance of a fellow human being. We select our partners to a large extend on the basis of how they look. That's because the visual impression is the easiest way to get information about another person. Furthermore, the advertising industry shamelessly exploits our visual instincts. We are manipulated by the charms of a youthful look. So we try for as long as possible to maintain the impression of being young.

Skin creams are still the most harmless products. They are not drugs. If they had any effect due to interacting with molecules inside our cells, they would have to be tested and approved as medicines. The main thing that skin creams do is to moisturize the skin and thus protect it from getting too dry. In this, skin creams perform a very useful function. Our skin is not designed to be washed daily with soap. Soap is a fantastic hygienic invention, as it effectively removes germs. But it dries the skin and makes it fragile; the loss of moisture makes the skin vulnerable to germs and damage. This is why it is recommended that we use skin cream. Anybody who is willing to invest in expensive anti-aging creams is not doing any harm, but cheaper, greasier skin creams help our skin just as much to endure the stress of daily washing.

Rigorous sun protection is important for the skin. The ultraviolet component of sunlight damages the DNA and can cause skin cancer as well as aging of the skin. Despite the complex DNA repair systems of human beings, a very specific and especially insidious kind of DNA damage remains in our skin cells. The UV-induced *cyclobutane-pyrimidine dimers*, CPDs for short, often go undetected and can lead to mutations that alter genetic information. CPDs are chemical compounds of two thymine bases, which interfere with the structure of the DNA. Only about twenty years ago several countries started introducing legislation banning teenagers from tanning studios. Until then particularly teenaged girls were keenly exposing themselves to dangerous UV radiation; and tanning studios remain popular with women under 25. They love the immediate tan, but they completely ignore the long-term life threatening danger. Skin cancer only develops decades later due to the effects of CPDs. These days we are beginning to see the consequences of the sun-seeking habits of the 1990s.

Human UV repair systems are still attuned to the times when our furry ancestors were far better protected from UV radiation. But there are also species that have been exposed to strong UV radiation for hundreds of millions of years. Algae and plants need to convert the energy of sunlight into biomass production, through photosynthesis. Marsupials such as kangaroos, which are close relatives of us placental mammals, are exposed to the sun's rays as young animals. These organisms must repair CPDs quickly and efficiently. To do this, they use a very simple enzymatic method. *CPD photolyase* is a very specialized protein that is designed only to recognize and repair CPDs. In contrast to the otherwise highly complex DNA repair systems, CPD photolyase is a single enzyme. Mice that carry a CPD photolyase from placental mammals are surprisingly well protected against UV-induced skin cancer [110].

Another enzyme that can repair CPDs particularly well is the T4 endonuclease 5. This enzyme comes from T4 bacteriophages, i.e., viruses that attack bacteria. There are sunscreens and skin creams available that contain CPD photolyase or T4 endonuclease V in liposomes. Liposomes are fat globules that can penetrate into the cells of the skin and thus can bring photolyase to where the DNA damage is. This method is not capable of completely repairing CPD damage, as the introduction of proteins by means of liposomes is not yet efficient enough, but it can help reduce the damage.

Even more important than repair is the consistent protection from UV radiation. Careless sun bathing, even in regions with relatively weak sunlight, is irresponsible. Even low-cost sunscreens provide some degree of protection. Nevertheless, it is essential to avoid exposing the skin to direct sunlight. Welcome as the warmth of the sun may be to those of us in the North, UV damage to our DNA remains a ticking time bomb for our health.

The rejuvenation of our outward appearance has become a profitable industry. Youthfulness is considered to be so desirable that Botox injections have become popular, and it's not only Hollywood actors who have their facial muscles paralyzed. And whether we're talking about Nicolas Cage, Silvio Berlusconi or Jürgen Klopp, hair transplants mask men's age better and better. Hereditary hair loss can also be delayed medically these days by inhibiting the steroid 5α-reductase. This prevents the conversion of the male sexual hormone testosterone into dihydrotestosterone, whereupon the growth activity of the hair follicles is increased. However, the youthful appearance only deceives us about the true age of the body, of course. It's far from clear that the external rejuvenation of an aging society is in fact a good thing.

The urge to look young is a form of denying that we are aging. We are already in the midst of a campaign purging the very signs and appearances of aging — but with an ever-increasing number of elderly, if we want to be a healthy society, we must protect ourselves from the negation of aging.

VI. Is There a Cure for Aging?

VI.1. Meteoric advances in modern medicine

Now let's talk about the impossibility of immortality, the return of the irrepressible scourge of humanity and the disease that is irrational human nature — for which we will never find a cure.

In the last twenty years our knowledge about aging has seen exponential growth. Never before has humankind known more about him- or herself. Never before has it been possible to treat diseases to this extent. We have learned from diverse biological model systems that under experimental conditions the life span can be extended and youth can be preserved longer. How do we use this knowledge for the benefit of human health? In the following chapter, new medical developments and therapies are explored. This time, we're not looking at cosmetic anti-aging products but potential therapies to combat real age-related diseases.

Looking at the wealth of knowledge now available thanks to modern gerontology research, we wonder whether drugs against "aging" may actually be at hand. But as the previous sections have made more than clear: aging is a complex process! All types of cells, tissues and organs must work every fraction of a second for our entire life span. Anyone who has been able to marvel at the fast opening and closing of the heart valves that cardiologists can visualize by ultrasound imaging inevitably asks how this might work for a whole lifetime. Our genetic blueprint is not adapted to preserving our body for an extended period after we pass our reproductive phase. In short, our body is not designed for eternity. Immortality is not achievable. But if not the life span, can we extend the quality of life?

This leads us to the way we age. One hundred years ago infectious diseases were still a major cause of death, and today about half the people in the developed world die of cardiovascular diseases — they succumb to a stroke or a heart attack. The second most common cause of death is cancer. Infectious diseases have been tamed, for the most part, since the development of vaccines, and have decreased considerably due to the work of the English physician and scientist Edward Jenner and the discovery of penicillin by the Scottish biologist Alexander Fleming. Humankind's victory over some of the worst infections is probably the greatest success in the history of medicine.

Certainly, we still have a long way to go before many of these diseases can be completely eradicated. Even polio, whose complete disappearance was already announced several times, has flared up again and again. Everyone is aware of how irresponsibly people can behave, from Pakistani Taliban who murder vaccination teams to fake news spread about the dire consequences of vaccinations in the US, or radical Christians who refuse to give their children access to modern medicine. Further, fatal and highly transmittable diseases such as HIV and tuberculosis are still running rampant. HIV is almost completely preventable. But this deadly virus is not capable of changing human behavior. At least, AIDS has been transformed into a treatable chronic disease through improved therapies. Tuberculosis, which has almost disappeared from our latitudes, is currently making a return.

Of particular concern are resistant strains that no longer respond to treatment. Flu bugs spread around the world with seasonal regularity. The Spanish flu claimed more victims in just one year than the entire First World War that was raging at the time. Bird flu hovers over us like a sword of Damocles, because no one can predict how severe it will be from year to year. Flu is transmitted by influenza viruses that can quickly change their genetic composition, thus evading recognition by our immune system.

Infectious diseases are always poised to make dangerous attacks on humanity. It's been a long time since infection research was ascribed the importance that it deserves, that much is clear. The Ebola epidemic, for instance, shows that we must not neglect vaccine research. In an era when even malaria could make a comeback in southern Europe, it seems easier to leave such research to philanthropists like Bill and Melinda Gates rather than shoulder our own social obligations to eradicate infectious diseases. No doubt, many medical (and political-social) steps have to be taken before we can tame these scourges of humanity. Nevertheless it is apparent that scientific and medical progress have fundamentally improved and extended the life of almost everyone — quite clearly in the West, but in the rest of the world as well.

VI.2. Disease prevention and therapy

Aging is not a disease and it is difficult to treat, especially since humans are convenience-seeking creatures and are so irrational that they would sit in a restaurant with a diesel engine running. But there are many contenders vying for positions among the leading causes of death.

For many of the ailments afflicting the elderly, we are close to being able to develop preventive therapies.

Since our body is not adapted to such advanced ages as we commonly reach these days, our cells and tissues can leave us in the lurch. Our immune system cannot keep up, either, and it can hardly protect us against even simple infections. Poorly functioning tissues can no longer maintain our bodily functions. Aging stem cells are no longer replaced on time. Wounds are difficult to heal. And one disease rarely comes alone in old age. Too many organs are affected. When the American demographer Jay Olshansky projected the effects on eliminating individual diseases on life expectancy, he realized that even spectacular leaps forward, such as a total victory over cancer would increase the average life expectancy of the population by merely 3 years. Other diseases — also age-related — are lurking on the list of top causes of death, and they would simply move up one position.

Prevention is better than treating a disease. Skin cancer is a striking example: It is hard to treat skin cancer, but it's relatively simple to cover the skin with clothes and sun block. That being said, prevention is more difficult with other types of cancer, and even skin cancer can occur independently of sunlight-inflicted damage.

Preventing a disease before it can occur is of course the best strategy. That is why vaccinations are such a blessing, because with a vaccine, we don't have to wait for an infectious disease to crop up. And a healthy lifestyle in itself can prevent diseases such as type 2 diabetes, while the risk of developing lung cancer can be dramatically reduced by not smoking.

As aging is by far the largest risk factor for cancer, dementia and physical deterioration, we need a comprehensive preventative therapy for the aging process itself. Aging can now be delayed in simple organisms. However, it is complicated to develop effective anti-aging therapies because of the fact that aging itself is not a disease. How can we develop a drug when there is no disease to treat? How would you know that a treatment has successfully prevented Alzheimer's? Epidemiological studies could show such an effect, but they take time and they need huge groups of subjects. This is why it is so important to develop meaningful biomarkers to monitor biological age. Such biomarkers would at least enable us to see the success of an anti-aging therapy.

One intervention that has produced impressive effects in many organisms, such as mice, not only in prolonging the life span but also in preventing aging-related diseases, is calorie restriction. Whether calorie restriction is conducive to health in humans, and whether it can extend our lives, is still under investigation. In the US, supporters of calorie restriction have joined together in the Calorie Restriction Society. Its members claim that the positive effects of calorie restriction have been proven. They are right in terms of prolonging the life of simple animals, but not of humans. As already discussed, the results on life span in primates are anything but clear, and even different mouse strains react quite differently to a reduced caloric intake. Radical self-experiments should be discouraged.

Obesity, on the other hand, must be combated. Obesity is an enormous risk to health. Overweight has become widespread even in health-conscious societies, and most alarmingly, among children and adolescents. The increase in life expectancy over the past 150 years might even come to a stop in the United States amid the widespread obesity. This represents a massive health problem for the time to come. A balanced diet is not self-evident. It takes a certain effort to manage our own food.

Like many aspects of the modern life style, the trend to eat out has spread from the US across the world. Fast food restaurants and take-out are part of our daily diet. Tacos and tortillas are no longer found only in big cities but in every little town and almost at every crossroads. Pizza and pasta, with cheap cheese and fatty sauces, fill you up at a low price. But even fast food burgers combine sugar and spices that induce a craving and make you thirsty, besides. Combined with greasy fries, many people consider this a whole meal. Instead of water, we rinse down our over-salted fast food with soft drinks and other over-sweetened chemical drinks that combine sugar and acids. And all of this is easy to find, no need to hunt for it — it's cheap, readily available, even at a gas station, and soon you want more.

It would take an enormous effort to radically change these modern eating habits. Cosmetic changes are not enough — things like an "alibi salad" in a fast food restaurant, served with a greasy sauce anyway because it simply tastes so much better and stimulates the desire for more. Even in restaurants, the portions are often larger than necessary. To cook for ourselves takes time and effort. Buying fresh ingredients is harder than picking up something ready-made. However, a healthy diet is essential if we want to keep our bodies healthy. Bad habits easily take hold. The desire for convenience is very human. To overcome it requires the insights of reason followed up by corresponding actions.

A healthy menu must also be put in place in cafeterias where a large part of the population eats every day. Even in the cafeteria of our University Clinic in Cologne, the line is always longest where the food is greasy and sweet instead of nutritious and healthy. The school lunchroom plays a very special role in the socialization of young people. To meet the requirements of limited public budgets, healthy nutrition, and the tastes of the students, we need to develop innovative nutrition concepts. This responsibility cannot be passed on to the authorities alone. We are responsible for our own family's food. And society has a common interest in ensuring that people have a healthy diet.

Former New York mayor Michael Bloomberg tried in vain to restrict the volume of soft drink containers to 16 ounces. At the movies, not only are soft drinks served in buckets that cost hardly more than smaller portions (16 ounces being the smallest size), but you can also refill your bucket as often as you like. In supermarkets as well, the prices for huge cola bottles are not much higher than for smaller bottles. When it comes to some things, unfortunately, the public's ability to use common sense and make rational decisions is so disappointing that it's hard to keep the state from intervening. Imposing smoking restrictions has greatly improved the environmental risks of office workers and restaurant waiters alike. Still, there are too many countries with lax regulations on public smoking. The argument that it should be up to the individual to decide where to smoke is simple, but then, you are not allowed to bring a diesel engine into a restaurant and poison the other guests. At home, every individual is free to be as unreasonable as he or she likes, and often the children of smoking parents are already exposed to the poison as infants.

Just as important as the food itself is how our body handles the food. Our metabolism changes early in life. After all, in the early stages of life the main thing is to absorb a lot of biomass so that your body can grow. Later the body must be maintained and tissue has to be replaced. In that phase, the biomass is utilized differently. We can see the difference for ourselves. When we are children, we literally "burn through" ice cream and sweets in great quantity without gaining weight, while as adults we easily put on pounds. Men may find themselves with either a "spare tire" or a beer belly; for women it is often the hips and thighs. Young bodies deal with fat differently than adults. Young people can consume fat efficiently, while already by middle age the fat just gets deposited.

The difference between the burning of fat and storage is due to the different composition of the adipose tissue. Brown fat cells are specialized for converting fatty acids to produce heat. The young body has plenty of brown fat cells. For a long time it was assumed that the adult body had no brown adipose tissue at all. In fact, the brown adipose tissue decreases as we age. In the adult body, the white fat cells predominate, and their main task is to store fat. If we could intervene to control the formation of brown and white fat cells, perhaps we could protect our bodies from getting fat.

Nutrition is only one part of a healthy lifestyle. Physical activity is perhaps even more crucial. Most of our 200,000 years of history as *Homo sapiens* was characterized by daily physical effort. Until our evolution to the "wise men" we were always running, climbing trees and running into physical confrontations with our own and other species; these were the main occupations.

The eight-hour day, spent sitting on a chair, is a modern practice for which our body was not designed. That is why we need to be physically active. Walking is the easiest and most straightforward way to keep the body in motion. But for us, that is often too time consuming. Yet regular physical activity may reduce the risk of cardiovascular disease significantly.

Strokes and heart attacks are still the leading causes of death. Each of us needs to adopt a clear prevention strategy, especially focusing on regular exercise. We should not give in to laziness. A stroke can be devastating. Life as we know it is usually totally disrupted. In serious cases, parts of the brain are permanently damaged and paralysis may leave the patient wheelchair bound or helpless in bed.

With heart attacks, the first few minutes before medical assistance arrives are crucial. Heart massages and resuscitation can be life-saving and any human being can do it. We should all be prepared to provide the right kind of assistance to help a victim quickly and efficiently.

For ourselves, it is essential to reduce the risk of cardiovascular disease through a healthy, physically active lifestyle. In addition, risks can often be detected at an early stage and, if necessary, cholesterol-lowering drugs can be prescribed.

VI.3. Cancer therapy: From a death sentence to a chronic disease

Learn how an air raid on an Italian port has saved thousands of lives so far, and look for the genetic Achilles heel of cancer cells to find out how and why intruders are recognized and driven out of our bodies on the basis of their ID cards.

The risk of developing cancer increases dramatically with age. Cancer is a highly complex disease and worse still, it is a disease of our own cells. The body has effective defense mechanisms against the formation of cancer, but again, our body has developed a defense that works very well while we are young but not so well in old age.

Although the "war on cancer" proclaimed by President Richard Nixon in the 1970s has not yet been won, we have made great progress in combating this highly complex disease. The realization that DNA damage can cause cancer has, in itself, made it possible to come up with measures for preventing cancer.

Most forms of skin cancer can be prevented by consistently protecting against UV rays. This presents more of a psychological hurdle than any practical obstacle for those in the north who like to spend their sun-drenched vacations indulging in irresponsible sunbathing.

The same applies to the enormous cancer risk caused by cigarette smoking. Here, the causative role of toxic substances in tobacco has been irrefutably proven for lung cancer and for a variety of other cancers and diseases as well. By avoiding smoking, we can prevent fatal diseases. While smoking in the United States is on the decline, cigarette smoking still ranks as the leading cause of preventable disease and death. Smoking still runs high among those who are economically deprived, with about a quarter of the poor and less-educated people exposing themselves to this hazard. It is not enough to call for better health care while taking such a high personal risk. To demand treatment for aging-related illnesses is almost ridiculous as long as one is not prepared to take better care of one's own body.

After all, by now everyone is aware of how much smoking damages our health. But nevertheless, people continue to talk calmly about their harmful nicotine consumption while avoiding recognizing that they are betraying themselves. Ultimately, smoking is an addiction. Cigarettes are not a pleasure, but a drug. Only the nicotine-addicted brain gives the impression that it is a free decision to light up another cigarette. The consciousness is manipulated by the nicotine receptors, which are addicted and want more ligands. This is precisely why social support is needed. Smoking is not a decision made by our free will, and quitting smoking requires addiction treatment. Most people develop their nicotine addiction when they are teenagers. Despite all the statements made by the tobacco industry, both their advertising and their products target this audience. Substances are added to the tobacco to suppress coughing and avoid irritating the taste buds of adolescents. They sell an image that appeals to teenagers. And being part of the group often means being a smoker.

Here, social action is necessary. In many countries, smoking bans have made the working environment, be it at the office, on an airplane, in a restaurant, or at a nightclub, significantly healthier. The widespread banishment of cigarettes from Hollywood movies may have contributed to the decline of smoking in the US. Smoking is now regarded as antisocial, and smokers are almost banned from the public. In this sense, American society has prevailed against the powerful tobacco industry.

In any case, cancer-causing substances must be eradicated from our environment. When the catalytic converter was introduced into motor vehicles in 1975, it soon became imperative to remove lead as a fuel additive (since it would destroy the converter). Now, if we ever come across an old car running on leaded fuel, we realize how polluted the cities must have been a few decades ago. Yet, industry at first resisted these changes, claiming it would drive up their costs.

The demand for diesel particulate filters set off the same defense mechanism on the part of the auto industry. Confidence in a corporate sense of responsibility (and not only in the auto industry) is seriously misplaced, as this example shows. Electric cars could significantly improve air quality in large cities; but that opens up a new set of questions, including how to assess the full environmental effects, which would include producing all that electricity as well as disposing of the batteries.

Short-term economic interests often prevent real progress. This is being played out in a dramatic fashion in China where millions of people have had their health ruined because even the simplest protective measures and environmental restrictions have not been permitted to hinder their economic development as they rush to modernize their vast country. The long-term cost for the people, who are often ill, but also for society, will be immeasurable. Long-term thinking, unfortunately, is not a human instinct.

It is extremely important that we prevent cancer, and there are, as described, some clear, even startlingly simple measures that people can take to reduce their own cancer risk. However, some tumors will occur even so. Because it is enough if even one single cancer cell is able to defeat all the checkpoints and all the efforts of the immune system and grow into a tumor. Once a tumor has formed, early detection is the first step in preventing it from developing into something worse.

Skin cancer can be recognized by the trained eye of the dermatologist at an early stage when, often, it is still harmless to remove it. But it is up to everyone to visit the dermatologist regularly. Other types of cancer require more or less invasive techniques to be recognized in the early stages. Breast cancer check-ups can give important indications during the initial scanning process. Mammograms are invasive, because they use radiation to image the breast tissue, and that in itself can also damage DNA. When a mammogram is advisable, it's best to ask your physician about this. Gastrointestinal cancer can be detected early by endoscopy. In men, prostate cancer testing may be advisable because this type of cancer occurs fairly often, but the existing test methodologies will require improvements to avoid unnecessary surgery.

As we have already seen in the chapter on DNA damage in cancer development, environmental influences and genetic factors both play an important role in determining our risk of cancer. Genetic factors are particularly important when certain types of cancer run in the family. Then it is particularly important to get tested on a regular basis. There are specific tests for certain risk-related mutations, such as the detection of mutations in the breast and ovarian cancer genes BRCA1 and BRCA2. It is hoped that such genetic tests will be offered at a lower cost in the future. In the meantime, the sequence of nucleotides for the whole genome can be determined for less than a $1,000.

But interpreting the data correctly is a far greater challenge than determining the sequence of an individual's genome. It is still far from simple to read one's risk of developing a specific type of cancer, or dementia, on the basis of a genome sequence. Ultimately, it is still largely unknown how the different variations of the genes interact with each other. Monogenic diseases, which are caused by the malfunction of just a single gene, are easy to diagnose. If someone carries a mutation in the BRCA genes, the cancer risk can be estimated relatively well. However, every person carries some variations in the approximately 25,000 human genes. A gene variant may have a different impact if the gene is surrounded by different variants of other genes. For reasons like this, the field of genetic diagnostics is still in its infancy. With the rapid development in the study of human genetics, diagnosis on the basis of genome sequencing should become an important predictive tool in the future.

But at the moment, despite improved early detection, cancer is still one of the deadliest diseases. Still, significant progress has been made in cancer therapy in recent years. For example, the rate of cures in childhood leukemia is now at seventy percent, thanks to radiotherapy. Like much in science, modern cancer therapy sprang from pure coincidence.

In December 1943, the American merchant ship S.S. *John Harvey* was bombed during a German air raid on the Italian port of Bari. On board the *John Harvey* there was a cargo that was as deadly as it was secret: mustard gas, a chemical that had been banned from the war because of the devastating atrocities it had caused in the previous world war. The cargo of mustard gas, one of the nitrogen mustards, polluted the surrounding areas after the bombardment. A short time later, while conducting autopsies, the doctors found the victims had a reduced white blood cell count. The attentive Italian doctors drew the correct conclusion: If the poison lowered the white blood cell count, it could be used to fight blood cancers. This laid the foundations for the development of chemotherapy.

Chemical substances that induce DNA damage will trigger the DNA damage checkpoints also in cancer cells, and thus they initiate the self-killing program called apoptosis. Although it took decades to investigate the effects of DNA damage, checkpoints and apoptosis, chemotherapy is widely used today, supplemented by radiation therapy (which uses ionizing radiation, which in turn causes DNA damage). Together with the surgical removal of cancerous tissues, this is the standard in treatment still today.

Naturally, chemical agents and irradiation can damage more than just the cancer cells. Cell types that grow and divide rapidly suffer the same fate as the cancer cells, because damage monitoring for the DNA is particularly active during cell division. That is why cells in the hair roots, the *hair follicles*, and those in the intestinal mucosa, the *intestinal epithelial cells*, also die — because both of them are constantly being renewed. This leads to hair loss and digestive disorders. The side effects of chemotherapy and radiotherapy can cause severe physical and emotional stress for the patient.

More modern therapies try targeting the cancer cells more specifically. In "personalized" therapy, efforts are made to find the genetic Achilles heel of the cancer cells. For example, if cancer cells carry a mutation in BRCA1, they malfunction when using recombination repair to fix double-strand breaks in the DNA. This is a very precise method for repairing double-strand breaks, using undamaged DNA as the basis for restoring the broken strand. In cells that lack functional BRCA1, the double-strand breaks have to be repaired by means of end-joining. If, however, this alternative repair mechanism is disabled by a specific drug, the cell is helplessly exposed to double-strand breaks. Such a drug that specifically inhibits the end-joining repair only works in cancer cells that carry a mutation in the BRCA1 gene, and is thus more efficient and has relatively low side effects.

However, even this tailor-made therapy is also subject to the adaptability of cancer cells. Cancer cells are very tolerant of the instability of their own genetic mutations and so they can accumulate further mutations. As a result, cancer cells develop resistance to therapies. Even though only a few cells survive after an initially successful therapy, in the next phase new mutations blunt the response to the same therapy. These surviving cancer cells divide over and over, and then grow into a therapy-resistant tumor.

One promising innovation in targeted therapy is antibody therapy. Here again, genetic mutations in the cancer cells are used. Each cell in the body presents itself to the immune system by displaying parts of its own proteins on the cell surface. The immune system recognizes these "identity cards" of its own inhabitants. If a mutation is present in a cell, this may lead to a change in the amino acid sequence of the proteins. The immune system can recognize this. Then the cell is no longer seen as an innocent citizen, but an intruder, and it is attacked as such.

Antibody therapy employs molecules of the adaptive immunity that recognize the unusual molecules on the surface of cancer cells and then alert the immune system to them. In doing so, our normal immune defense is used to destroy cancer cells, without the normal, healthy cells being affected as they are in chemotherapy and radiotherapy. Immunotherapy in particular offers a great opportunity to convert cancer into a chronic disease with which one can lead a normal life while undergoing therapy.

The total eradication of cancer cells appears to be rather unrealistic, since the survival of even individual cancer cells is enough to go on and form a dangerous tumor later on. But for now, we have not yet reached the goal of eliminating the deadly risk of cancer. Because cancer is a disease of our own cells, because so many different mutations can lead to cancer, and because, due to the instability of the genome, each cancer cell can be genetically different, cancer therapy remains one of the greatest medical challenges.

VI.4. The requirements for anti-aging treatments

Better young, beautiful and dead or old but still alive? We need to find out why we age, in order to survive!

In the future, cancer will be a particular challenge for anti-aging therapies. The hormonal shifts that occur during aging lead to a reduction in cell growth. This makes it harder to regenerate tissues, as the stem cells become less active.

The diminished activity of the signaling pathway that originates from the messenger IGF-1 prolongs the life of roundworms, fruit flies and mice. This pathway also controls the growth of the body, which is why the long-lived Snell and Ames mice remain dwarfish — because the IGF-1 signaling pathway stimulates cell division and thus growth. Reducing it can stop the growth not only of normal cells, it also stops the growth of cancer cells. Age-related hormonal shifts, away from body growth to simply maintaining the tissues, are the body's attempt to survive despite increased DNA damage. Reduced activity of the growth hormones and IGF-1 in response to accumulating DNA damage is an example of this. So you could say that we age in order to survive! Hormonal therapies can be used, as we shall see, to rejuvenate tissues. However, they always carry the risk of promoting the growth of cancer cells at the same time. For this reason, the success of future anti-aging therapies will depend on the effective control of cancer.

So, we see that the main causes of death in our population can already be reduced by exercising clear prevention strategies, and also by using improved therapies. However, even with a healthy lifestyle, these diseases will not be completely avoided. Preventive measures such as healthy eating and regular physical activity can effectively reduce the risk of cardiovascular disease and type 2 diabetes. Some risk factors can be avoided; but there are other factors that we can less easily influence.

Cancer is one of the most complex diseases in the world and it cannot be fully understood nor adequately treated even after decades of the greatest scientific efforts. However, impressive successes have already been recorded in the treatment of even complicated cancer types. In the meantime, cancer therapy can significantly increase the life expectancy of many patients. As we identify more individually-tailored, "precision medicine" therapies, even resistant cancer cells may be attacked and lead to the success of treatment where hitherto little hope existed. In such cases, cancer could become a chronic but tolerable disease.

VI.5. Treatment Approaches for Age-Related Dementia

Now to Aubrey de Grey, the engineer of the aging brain, who was looking for human spare parts in the graveyard and found microbes. In addition, a few words on treating Alzheimer's disease and the associated danger of decaying while we're still alive.

There is still a great deal of uncertainty about the causes of age-related dementia and how treatable it may be. After the age of eighty-five, nearly one in two people suffer from dementia. However, there is as yet no effective therapy that would enable us to effectively fight or prevent dementia such as Alzheimer's. The gradual diminution in brain function is one of the reasons that old age is still invariably associated with serious disease.

Scientific research in the field of age-related dementia has led to a much better understanding of the causes and progression of Alzheimer's and Parkinson's disease. Parkinson's patients suffer particularly from the loss of nerve cells that produce the messenger dopamine. The therapeutic use of dopamine or deep brain stimulation can compensate for this loss and help patients regain control of their muscles.

Restoring the nerve cells that produce dopamine would, of course, be far more desirable than simply taking dopamine supplements or achieving electrical signal enhancement through electrodes. An example of such a treatment concept is seen with Parkinson's patients, where this type of nerve cells may be introduced into the brain to replace the dead cells and take over the function of dopamine production. At the moment, the goal is to create new nerve cells from stem cells, which can then take over the production of dopamine in Parkinson's patients.

Alzheimer therapy presents even greater challenges to medical research. It is not yet entirely clear what the main factors of this disease are. The plaques formed by beta-amyloid peptides in the patient are also said to have protective functions. Apparently it is not the large clumps of plaques themselves but rather the oligomers, that is, the accumulation of just a few misfolded beta-amyloid molecules that bring on the disease.

Breaking down beta-amyloid is an important therapeutic concept. The British gerontologist and author Aubrey de Grey, who is more known from the media than from the literature, has devised a proposal that is convincing in its simplicity. De Grey is a trained computer scientist whose approach is that of the engineer's. De Grey runs the "SENS Foundation," supported by private sponsors, and he promises a radical life extension. According to him, soon we will be able to live ten thousand years. In the end, just like with an old car, body parts always need repairs. To that end, De Grey has been looking for substances that can break down beta-amyloid plaques. And where, at the end of the day, are patients' plaques completely broken down? You guessed it; de Grey went to the cemetery to find the microbes that digest the human body while it's decaying. De Grey succeeded and suggested a most simple therapy concept for Alzheimer's disease. However, how the bacterial digestion enzymes would be tailored to specifically degrade beta amyloid and not instead decay patients who are still alive remains to be sorted out.

More realistic approaches stem from knowledge of natural protein degradation mechanisms. Here, much hope is placed in autophagy as the natural way to dissolve larger protein clumps.

The first substances to boost autophagy have already been isolated. Polyamines such as spermidine — a protein, which, despite its name, is found not only in sperm but in animals, plants and fungi — are currently being tested to stimulate autophagy. Frank Madeo, a researcher in Graz, Austria, initially administered spermidine to flies, then roundworms and mice, and it extended the life span in all three [111]. Together with Stephan Sigrist from the Free University of Berlin, Madeo even delayed age-related decline of memory function in flies by using spermidine [112].

Rapamycin and caloric restriction also stimulate autophagy and may make a therapeutic contribution in treating Alzheimer's. However, patients with advanced Alzheimer's disease are likely to be at risk of nutritional deficiencies and they need regular meals. Careful clinical testing is also imperative; so far, animal models show promising results. Precisely because caloric restriction lends itself so easily to self-testing, we need clear clinical data to prove that the advantages outweigh the side effects. Conceptually, scientists are currently trying to identify the active substances that put the body in the caloric restriction state without the food actually being reduced. One such substance is rapamycin, which as discussed earlier inhibits the TOR complex. However, as we have already learned, it has not been proven that caloric restriction extends the life span in primates. In addition, rapamycin leads to immunosuppression; it lowers our immune defense. Such treatment might therefore leave our bodies defenseless against attacks from pathogens.

We already know that reducing IGF-1 activity can lead to a longer life for simple nematode worms, flies and mice, although the situation is already somewhat more complicated in mice. A complete lack of the IGF-1 receptor prevents even embryonic growth. No one wants to change places with a Laron syndrome patient whose growth hormone receptor does not work.

Could a targeted shutdown of IGF-1 activity in adults be successful? Inhibitors against IGF-1 activity have already been developed by many pharmaceutical companies. But they were not concerned about using it against aging. The growth of cancer cells is also often controlled by IGF-1. Therefore, IGF-1 inhibitors have been clinically tested to see if they can prevent cancer growth, even if no resounding clinical success has been achieved so far.

But there is yet another interesting observation that has been made in mice that form only small amounts of the IGF-1 receptor. Andrew Dillin in California and Markus Schubert in Cologne investigated such mice in an Alzheimer model [113], [114]. Nerve cells that lacked the gene for the IGF-1 receptor were protected from the clumping of beta-amyloid peptides. Despite an Alzheimer's mutation in the amyloid precursor protein, APP, the nerve cells were protected from Alzheimer's disease because the IGF-1 receptor was not active. It is therefore conceivable that specific inhibition of IGF-1 activity has a positive effect in Alzheimer's disease.

However, deactivating IGF-1 across the board could compromise the body's regenerative capacity. That's because IGF-1 is important for stimulating cell growth, including that of stem cells. Thus, IGF-1 based therapy should be targeted to specific cell types, such as nerve cells that never have to divide. Otherwise, severe side effects could occur in other tissues, such as the blood system or the intestine, as these tissues depend on a high rate of regeneration.

VI.6. Stem Cells and Regenerative Medicine

In this chapter you will find a recipe for stem cells (warning: may contain traces of cancer), sewing instructions for mice, and a few facts about a frog that proved the dogma of cell differentiation.

A successful anti-aging therapy must not only maintain existing tissues (which is crucial for nerve cells which, once they are formed, are never replaced) but also bring about the ongoing regeneration of aged tissue. Some tissues regenerate all the time, for example the skin and intestines. Both are constantly growing, as the outer layers of the cells are exposed to severe hazard. Stem cells are responsible for regenerating these layers. Through cell division, stem cells can bring forth new cells, which can then develop into specialized skin or intestinal cells. The number of these stem cells is limited and in some stem cell compartments, such as the muscles, their number decreases during aging. But it is not just decreasing numbers; the older the stem cells are, the less capable they are to give rise to the whole range of specialized cells that are required to replenish tissues.

This has been observed especially in the bone marrow, where the blood cells are formed in adult humans. The red blood cells that supply our cells with oxygen live only up to 120 days maximum. Some white blood cells live just a few days. Our blood cells must therefore be constantly renewed. We used to think that the number of stem cells would decrease with age.

Gerald de Haan and Gary Van Zant traced stem cells as they aged, to measure their ability to form blood cells in mice. To their astonishment, they found that old mice had by no means fewer stem cells in their bone marrow [115]. However, the old stem cells could no longer form the different blood cell types to the same extent as young stem cells. So it's not the number of stem cells in bone marrow that decreases with age, but their ability to form certain types of blood cells. Transplanting young stem cells, however, was shown to improve the blood count.

Stem cell therapy is already used in cancer treatment. Leukemia patients have to be treated with high doses of ionizing radiation or chemotherapeutic agents — which damage the genome of the cells and lead to cell death in the rapidly dividing cancer cells. Normal blood cells are also destroyed. The stem cells in the bone marrow in particular suffer greatly from this treatment. If, however, a suitable donor is found, the cancer patient's blood system can be restored by transplanting healthy bone marrow.

It is therefore quite conceivable that stem cell therapies could renew aging tissue. Particularly interesting observations have been made by the cell biologist and physician Thomas Rando at Stanford University in recent years. Rando is particularly interested in muscle regeneration. When muscles are injured, damage occurs to muscle cells, which must be replaced. To repair muscles, stem cells are activated, which renew the muscle tissue.

The regenerative capacity of the muscles decreases with age. Which factors are responsible for this decrease is not exactly known. Stem cells, however, need growth factors to activate their cell division and form new cells.

When a stem cell divides, it produces another stem cell and a second, precursor cell from which specialized cells such as muscle or intestinal cells are derived. Stem cells divide far less frequently than precursor cells. The precursor cells are used as much as possible in the construction and maintenance of tissues. The stem cells, instead, are protected. Every time the cells divide, there is a risk to the integrity of the genome of the cell.

During replication, when a copy of the genome is made before the cell divides, errors and thus mutations can occur. Cell division may result in an unequal distribution of chromosomes, that is, *aneuploidy*. So the body protects its stem cells by giving the main task of cell division to the precursor cells.

Stem cells can divide equally (symmetrically) or unequally (asymmetrically). In the case of symmetrical division, two cells are formed, either two stem cells or two precursor cells. External signals will determine the fate of the cells. If one of the cells leaves the stem cell niche, it loses the properties of a stem cell and becomes a precursor cell. For asymmetric division, one cell remains a stem cell while the sister cell becomes a precursor cell.

Stem cells, however, do not just decide to divide on their own. Their division is guided by growth factors. As the body ages, less growth factor is produced. Some growth factors are produced centrally, such as the growth hormone that is formed in the pituitary gland. Other growth factors, such as IGF-1, will be produced in various body parts such as the liver. Growth factors can act locally, on the surrounding cells, or they can be transported through the bloodstream and then exert their effect to distant tissues.

In order to study the significance of the growth factors circulating in the bloodstream, Rando together with Irina and Michael Conboy had a simple and ingenious idea. They stitched young and old mice together and thus connected their circulatory systems. This is called *heterochronic parabiosis*, to describe the connected lives of the animals of different age. The result was astonishing: Suddenly, the muscles of the old mice could regenerate as if they were young. Rando and the Conboys had succeeded in rejuvenating the muscles by connecting an old animal to a young bloodstream [116].

Building on Rando's findings, Amy Wagers continued to search for the growth factors that were the decisive factors in this rejuvenation effect. Wagers identified the growth differentiation factor GDF11, which decreases in aging mice and can be returned to them from the circulatory system of the younger mammals. When Wagers injected the GDF11 protein directly into old mice, the muscle tissue was rejuvenated [117]. The discovery of this type of rejuvenating factors in young blood opens up entirely new possibilities in regenerative therapy. Now it is conceivable that targeted use of growth factors such as Wagers GDF11 can be used to restore aging tissues. Whether eventually this will be as simple as using a single growth factor or rather requires a combination of several ones remains to be sorted out.

Stem cell therapies could indeed be applicable in the near future in diseases like muscular dystrophy. Regenerative medicine will play a central role in the prevention of aging-related diseases. But there are still great hurdles to overcome. If growth factors are used, as in Wager's experiments, we have to find a way to control the associated cancer risk.

Blood stem cells can be isolated decades in advance and can be delivered via bone marrow transplant to recipients whose own blood stem cells, called *hematopoietic stem cells*, have been killed by radiation therapy to control cancer. Stem cells can be recognized and concentrated on the basis of characteristic markers on their surface. It is relatively simple to derive stem cells from bone marrow. Other stem cells are much harder to access.

The stem cell therapy of the future will be highly dependent on whether the required stem cells can be obtained and delivered to patients whose own stem cells are no longer adequately functioning. The different cell types in our bodies, whether nerve cells, liver cells, various types of blood cells, bone and cartilage cells, or others, differ in their function and appearance, but they all carry the same copy of our genome. (Strictly speaking, two copies. Very strictly speaking, every copy of the genome is just slightly different because mutations can crop up when DNA is being copied during cell division.)

A stem cell has completely different properties than a specialized cell, or, to say it in professional jargon, a *differentiated* cell — say, a muscle cell; however, the two cell types still contain the same genome in their nucleus. Normally, stem cells differentiate only in one direction. Like Crick's central dogma of molecular biology, DNA makes RNA makes protein, and the corresponding dogma of cell differentiation is: Stem cells make precursor cells make differentiated cells. But just like with Crick's central dogma, where there are rules, there are exceptions. The British development biologist John Gurdon had already made a striking discovery in the 1950s. Gurdon took the cell nucleus with the genome contained in it from a frog's body cell and transplanted it into an emptied-out oocyte or egg cell, and from this a whole frog grew [118]. Gurdon thus proved that the genome of a body cell can be reprogrammed and can produce any other cell type, even a whole animal.

One of the biggest breakthroughs in stem cell research was achieved by Kazutoshi Takahashi and Shinya Yamanaka, of Japan, who discovered transcription factors (proteins that determine how genes are used) that can reprogram differentiated cell types, such as skin cells, into stem cells [119], [120]. These stem cells are called *induced pluripotent stem cells*, iPSC for short. "Pluripotent" describes the property that enables these cells to form many other cell types. While Dolly, the cloned sheep, was produced when the nucleus of a body cell was implanted in an egg cell to make a new animal using the genome of the donor, Takahashi and Yamanaka only needed to introduce the four genes *Oct3/4*, *Sox2*, *Klf4* and *Myc* into a body cell to convert it into a pluripotent cell. In this way, theoretically, an unlimited number of stem cells are available for stem cell therapy, and they can be generated from the patient's very own cells.

However, attentive readers will not have missed the fact that Myc is also an oncogene, a gene that fuels cancer growth. Myc activity can cause cancer. Moreover, it's no trivial matter to introduce genes into a patient. In the end, the stem cell factors have to be switched off in order to allow the stem cells to differentiate into the desired cell types. To this end, the reprogramming cocktail of the four genes has now been improved so that the genes will stay active for just a short time, and they are switched off again after they succeed in reprogramming the differentiated cells into stem cells.

Once stem cells have been obtained, they can also be turned into different cell types by the addition of specific compositions of growth factors and hormones. In theory, all cell types can be obtained in this way. The idea of using stem cell therapy to treat genetic diseases is particularly interesting; that is, to help a patient who has a mutation in a particular gene. In the stem cells a gene defect can be remedied, and then the healthy cells can be used in the patient. It is conceivable that stem cell therapy will soon enable us to restore stem cell tissue and thus repair and rejuvenate aging tissues.

But it is not only the stem cells that determine whether a tissue can be regenerated. The endocrine environment, that is, the growth factors circulating in the blood, play a decisive role. This was demonstrated by Thomas Rando's *parabiosis* experiments as well as the studies on prematurely aging mice that lacked the gene for *Sirt6* or that had shortened telomeres and therefore could not form blood by hematopoietic stem cells. Successful stem cell therapy will have to be embedded in endocrine rejuvenation, for example through the targeted use of growth factors.

VI.7. The magic pill

The path to longevity runs through a cask of red wine; or what we can learn from what was supposedly the first pill for eternal youth, the beneficial effects of the enzyme Sirtuin 1, and the fight against multimorbidity.

The anti-aging strategies discussed so far take into account the complexity of the aging process in humans by combining a variety of approaches. The diversity of our body tissues suggests, first and foremost, that a nerve cell threatened by Alzheimer's needs a different treatment than a stem cell that regenerates. In cancer therapy, individualized treatment goes one step further by following a tailor-made therapy for every cancer.

As we grow older, we become ill more often and more severely. The immune system is weaker in fighting off infections, bones break even upon minor impact, and the risk of developing cancer goes up dramatically. You could say that aging seems to be a common cause of various diseases, whether dementia, most forms of cancer, or cardiovascular diseases. All our tissues lose some functionality as we get older, whether we are talking about the lungs, kidneys, liver, muscles or bones.

Evolutionary biology has already explained to us why bodily functions decline and we are at a greater risk of getting sick. Our own evolutionary history has selected our genes so that our body will be at its best until the genes have been passed on to the next generation. Once the progeny has been generated, the further survival of the parents is no longer necessary for the evolutionary success of the species. Humans are still given a post-reproductive grace period, because it takes children a long time to learn all the vital knowledge they need from their parents, and because even grandparents — at least grandmothers — increase the reproductive success of their children and thus they help ensure that the genes continue to be passed on.

But can there be a "magic pill" that could stop the aging process as a whole? Some gerontology researchers are convinced that, any day now, an anti-aging pill will revolutionize medical practice. Instead of treating individual aging-related diseases, the problem will be tackled at the root. According to this view, arresting the aging process should prevent many serious diseases from setting in.

Are we just about to hit on the recipe for the long-awaited fountain of youth, or are these expectations exaggerated or just pipe dreams? The results in models using simple organisms suggest that this kind of all-encompassing therapy could indeed be near at hand. A single mutation in the *daf-2* gene is all it takes to double the life span of the roundworm. The critter remains agile and healthy for far longer. Rapamycin, the substance that disables the TOR complex, prolonged the lifespan of mice in a large-scale study even though the treatment was begun only at the age of 270 days, that is, long after the mice reached adulthood [69]. In the meantime, attempts are being made to develop more specific inhibitors that will have an effect similar to rapamycin — but without the negative effects of suppressing the immune system. Unless rapamycin proves to exert sufficient health-promoting effects at doses that are low enough so that the immune defense is not compromised, this drug has to be counted out as an anti-aging treatment in humans. Whether this can be achieved remains to be seen.

David Sinclair, an Australian researcher at Harvard University, is probably one of the most fervent supporters of the idea of the anti-aging pill. He has set his mind on using the enzyme sirtuin 1 as a therapy target. Based on their landmark studies of aging in baker's yeast, Guarente and Sinclair have developed sirtuin into an anti-aging weapon. Sirtuin can stop the aging of the yeast cells by preventing the formation of circular DNA sections that are toxic to the yeasts and therefore limit their lifespan [9]. Although this type of circular DNA structures do not occur in other species, sirtuin activity was found to have a life-prolonging effect a little later in roundworms and fruit flies [121], [122]. Mice, like humans, possess seven sirtuin genes, which act in different cell compartments. They are also credited with having positive effects on cell metabolism and on the stability of the genome. Also, the enzyme sirtuin helps keep the inner clock going, which ensures that the processes of our body are in sync with the natural circadian (day-and-night) rhythm.

Shortly after the turn of the millennium, Konrad Howitz came across resveratrol, a vegetable polyphenol that activates sirtuin. Sinclair then fed baker's yeasts with the sirtuin activator, and in fact the cells did live longer [123]. Sinclair assumed that resveratrol put the cells into the caloric restriction state and achieved its life-prolonging effects that way. Resveratrol did not prolong the life expectancy of mice, but when Sinclair fed obese mice high amounts of resveratrol, they fared much better. They survived longer than the overweight control group [124].

Resveratrol is a plant substance found in raspberries, plums, peanuts and, in different quantities, in red wine (grapes) too. The media naturally jumped on this connection. Suddenly everyone had a scientifically-based justification for drinking red wine. And in large quantities, because in order to get enough resveratrol to come anywhere near to having any effect, you would basically have to get wasted on red wine every day.

In addition, resveratrol only stays in the bloodstream very briefly, because it is immediately disposed of in the liver. So better, more specific and more stable sirtuin agonists were needed. *Agonist* (from Greek *agonististes* = "the agent") is the name for substances that increase the activity of a molecule, in this case a substance that would increase the potency of sirtuin. And drugs had to be made from molecules. To this end Sinclair, together with Christoph Westphal, founded Sirtris Pharmaceuticals, Inc.

Since aging in itself is not a disease, the idea was that Sirtuin agonists should first be used to prevent or treat diabetes and cancer. According to this plan, many people would quickly be able to activate their sirtuins to protect themselves from type 2 diabetes and cancer as typical age-associated diseases. Later, we can always see if Sirtris' drugs could also protect against Alzheimer's or even delay aging.

The potential of sirtuin agonists caught the attention of GlaxoSmithKline, and the pharmaceutical giant bought Sinclair's and Westphal's company for $720 million. But soon they came to doubt the efficacy of resveratrol and the other sirtuin agonists developed by Sirtris. Competing pharmaceutical companies Amgen and Pfizer tested Sirtris' compounds and did not find either resveratrol or other sirtuin agonists to be effective [125], [126].

Probably the different results are due to the fact that they used different versions of the sirtuin protein to test the activating effect of the agonists. While Sirtris used a version of sirtuin that was marked with a dye, the competition used the sirtuin protein as it is naturally found in the cell. In the meantime, sirtuin's life-prolonging effect has also been questioned in several organisms. David Gems in London reported that increasing the amount of sirtuin failed to increase the lifespan in roundworms and fruit flies [127]. After this report, new data were published that showed a significant, albeit relatively small, extension of the life span when the sirtuin content was elevated.

Sirtuins are certainly important proteins that are involved in various biological processes.[1] They help the cell in measuring the energy level, and they promote the stability of the genome and the metabolism of the mitochondria.[2] Research activity on sirtuins remains intense and modulating sirtuin activity might well play an important role in future anti-aging treatments. It remains to be seen whether the use of specific agonists to increase sirtuin activity can help fight the effects of aging in humans.

Even though there might not be a "magic pill" against aging, it is important to prevent or at least delay the onset of age-related diseases by extending health span. Israeli-born Nir Barzilai once served as a medical officer during the Entebbe raid that freed over one hundred hostages from the hands of Idi Amin, and later as a doctor he helped refugees at the Cambodian border, before he shifted his focus to the treatment of aging. At the Albert Einstein College of Medicine in New York, Barzilai is leading the "Target Aging with Metformin" (TAME) study that aims to determine whether metformin might

1 Sirtuins modify proteins by removing an acetyl group. Similar to phosphorylation, the activity of proteins can also be regulated by acetylation. Deacetylation, the removal of acetyl groups from other proteins by sirtuins, depends on the metabolic status of the cell because the sirtuins use the "energy chip," NAD.

2 Just like other types of modifications, whether phosphorylation, methylation, sumoylation or ubiquitinylation, which alter the properties of proteins by adding phosphate, methyl, sumo or ubiquitin groups, sirtuin-controlled acetylation is also used to regulate proteins.

confer anti-aging properties in humans. Metformin seems to mimic the effects of calorie restriction and has been used for treating type-2 diabetes for several decades. The effects of metformin on improving health in those people have encouraged researchers to run a larger trial to verify positive effects on reducing risk for age-related diseases including cardiovascular diseases and cancer.

The TAME study is particularly important for persuading the US Food and Drug Administration (FDA) to establish aging as an indication that could be targeted by a drug. Such an indication could then inspire the pharmaceutical industry to invest in the development of anti-aging drugs.

Aging as a clinical indication could be determined by the occurrence of age-related diseases in the form of multimorbidity, i.e., when a person suffers from at least two chronic diseases at the same time. Multimorbidity increases rapidly after the age of 60; over half of the people beyond the age of 65 suffer from at least two chronic diseases simultaneously. A better definition of biomarkers that allow the assessment of disease risk and biological age will in the future facilitate clinical trials for effective anti-aging treatments. Future treatments must target the aging process itself as only by extending health span it will be possible to prevent the variety of age-related diseases that often occur in combinations.

The search for anti-aging therapies is a major endeavor that is necessary for tackling age-related diseases. The first pioneering approaches have focused on targets that are involved in responses to calorie restriction, as this regime has proven to extend life span and to promote health in a variety of animals. Such therapeutic concepts aim at conferring the benefits of calorie restriction in a controlled way without necessarily altering food intake or eating habits. It is important to keep in mind that we are witnessing the very first clinical translations of the insights that were gained after just two decades of modern aging research.

Treating aging is an entirely novel concept for medical therapies. Thus far, researchers have focused on treating individual diseases once they occur. Given the pioneering character of these drug developments, occasional failure will be inevitable on the path to novel types of medical breakthroughs. We should not be discouraged but instead learn, particularly from those trials that might not have brought the desired success. It is imperative to find effective treatments that extend health span and prevent age-related diseases if we want to live in a healthy aging society in the future.

VII. THE OUTLOOK: THE FUTURE OF THE AGING SOCIETY

Even without breakthrough medical developments in cancer therapy or age-related dementia, even without the "magic anti-aging pill," we are getting older. Every seven years we gain an additional year. Newborns today have good prospects of living to the age of one hundred. This increased life expectancy is certainly a great achievement of civilization.

Living in our era, at least in the prosperous West, would probably seem to our ancestors like living in paradise. Until we reach our mid-30s, that is, the average life expectancy of people in the Middle Ages, most of us are free of serious illness. Even the poorest among us do not go without food, and the worst living standards are not remotely comparable to what was until just a few centuries ago the norm for the majority of the population.

But even when the aging of society presents us with such huge challenges, we should never forget in what happy times we were born into. Never have we had infectious diseases so much under control, never before have we known so much about the inner workings of the world and what keeps it all going, never before have the freedom of thought and action been possible that today we take for granted.

But our life is not youth everlasting, the way the daily flood of advertising and TV programs portray it. Sooner or later, all of our lives will show the imprint of aging. Those who are younger have to take care of their elders; it was always thus. It used to be primarily a family matter. Having a lot of children meant not only family happiness, but safety and security when people reach an age where they can no longer fend for themselves.

Since the Industrial Revolution, the traditional model of the family care largely vanished. More recently, public structures have had to be created to provide care for the old and the ill. In most of Europe, caring for the sick and the elderly has become a challenge for society as a whole. Even in more individualistic societies such as the United States, where traditionally preference has been given to "liberty" rather than the power of the state and any socialist or "collective" frameworks are viewed skeptically, it is increasingly recognized that society as a whole has a responsibility for the poor and the weak. This idea is not based entirely on charity. German Chancellor Otto von Bismarck astutely recognizing in the late 1880s that sick workers are not productive workers, and that they need rest and medical care in order to return to the workforce. He introduced the first state-run social benefit program.

The system works well as long as there are enough people to care for the old and the ill. In the 1950s, people lived an average of nine years after retirement. Meanwhile, however, the average person is living twice as long on their pension benefits. However, the working life span has changed little. We are in the midst of demographic change. As the baby boomers start reaching retirement age, a smaller number of young people will have to care for an ever-expanding proportion of elderly. By 2030, in many European countries including Germany, a third of the population will be over 65. This trend is slower in the United States due to slightly higher birth rates and immigration, but by then every fifth citizen will be above 65 years of age. By the year 2060, men's average life expectancy is projected to be 85 years, and for women it is nearly 90. Nowhere in the world is the demographic change affecting a society more rapidly and profoundly than in China. Increased life expectancy combined with the one-child policy that was introduced in the 1970s will result in about 500 million elderly among the projected 1.5 billion Chinese in 2050. The increase in life expectancy is not affecting developed countries alone. Instead, by 2050 about 1.5 of the 2 billion elderly in the world will live in less developed regions.

In just a few years, every two workers will have to cover the costs of one pensioner. As the baby boomer generation goes into retirement, we see that they produced fewer children. Given a birth rate of about 1.8 children per woman in the US and 1.6 in China, the population is inevitably shrinking. In many European countries, the birth rate is even lower, significantly so, and in the US it is mainly the high birth rate of the Latinos that keeps the population from shrinking faster. In rural areas, the social structures are giving way as so few young people have remained and they become outnumbered by the elderly.

Is this a taste of things to come? The demographic trend is indisputable and cannot be ignored. National pension systems are dying a slow death. The funding base for Social Security is at risk. IRAs, annuities, and other private retirement mechanisms will help some. But when we take the demographic decline into consideration, it is clear that our current pension programs need radical reforms. This trend is a tidal wave coming straight at us.

But the most comfortable way to deal with challenges that seem overwhelming is to simply ignore them. It is one of our basic instincts to stick with what is comfortable. Fear of losing what we have overpowers any hope of what we may achieve. If a politician wants to win, he or she has to convince the majority — but few people are willing to try something new. When people think they are at risk of losing something, they begin to fight; and if necessary, they may insist that the retirement age should not go up — in fact, maybe they'd like to see it even lowered — no matter what the demographic facts might project. The right to retire after as many years of labor as generations before us speaks directly to our feeling of social and economic justice.

We should, however, not forget that people's socio-economic situation plays an important part in determining life span and the propensity of suffering from age-related disease. A study in the Dutch region around Groningen showed that the lowest quarter of income earners lived on average seven years shorter and developed age-related diseases fourteen years earlier in comparison to the top 25% of income earners. Similarly a study in the UK revealed a dramatically shorter life expectancy of people living in poor as compared to wealthy regions. It certainly is neither the money alone nor genetic effects that make the economically deprived regions hot spots of early onset of diseases. Instead, the data suggest that interventions for healthy aging, such as healthy diet and physical activity, would produce the most profound benefits to the economically least privileged members of our society. But healthy aging also demands that retirement age should take into account the individual's biological age and the personal risk for developing age-related diseases, not only his or her chronological age.

The demographic shift requires dramatic changes and instead of defending the status quo, we need to adjust the way our economy runs. Productivity cannot be limited to a shrinking section of working-age people in an ever-aging society. Wealth is related to productivity, and productivity is dynamic. America's GDP is not simply the value of all the raw materials used, "the sum of all its parts" — we need to take into account how much value is added by transforming materials through engineering. We always need innovative, creative ideas and a social environment that is prepared to implement new ideas into innovations. Many ground-breaking inventions, from the toothbrush to the internal combustion engine, were produced by clever people working in small workshops or even only by pure coincidence, such as Alexander Fleming's penicillin. Science and innovation come from unexpected ideas and careful observation. But innovation and inventions can only thrive in a fertile environment. Inertia is their worst enemy.

And we will not be able to sustain the current standard of living simply by increasing the population, at this point. Even if the birth rate goes up in some miraculous way, it will take a massive investment in day care centers, schools, vocational and higher education institutions and universities for the next thirty years to eventually see a larger number of working people that could cover the costs of the growing army of retirees.

Some European countries including Germany promote a tax structure designed to help families with children through subsidized day care and tax breaks, a concept that has recently gained significant support, particularly among young people, in the United States as well. This "family" policy, however, is actually a disguised population policy, i.e., it aims to encourage a higher birth rate. In this regard, however, it has failed spectacularly. Perhaps the one-sided discussion of the issue, focusing primarily on the financial aspects, has only stoked potential parents' fears as they contemplate the burdens of starting a family. That being said, there is a limit to the role government can properly play. Family planning is better left to the parents, while the state (together with the employers who benefit from the professional activity of the parents) provide a functioning infrastructure.

Decades of low birth rates produce effects that cannot be reversed any time soon. Therefore the growth or decline of population needs to be handled separately from the question of how to support our aging society. Immigration, of course, is also being used to boost the number of working-age people.

To maintain their existing population numbers, immigration will have to account for at least 25% in many European countries. The wealthy country of Switzerland is leading the charge in this. The prosperity of this alpine country is based to a large extent on immigration. This is particularly true in the field of elder care, but it also applies to the field of research. Swiss research and innovation is indeed quite reliant on foreign scientists.

However, immigration is highly controversial. In Switzerland, and even in the United States with recent examples of xenophobia against a growing Latino population, there is a great deal of confusion. Between the extremes of multiculturalism and the desire to be tolerant and accepting of diversity, on the one hand, and a denial of the effects of runaway immigration on the other, there has been little chance of a rational discussion.

The U.S. and Canada, founded as nations of immigrants, have been dealing with this for longer than the more traditional European nations, but even there, the more liberal immigration policies since the 1980s have challenged social cohesion. Particularly people who feel themselves disadvantaged in society feel threatened by immigrants even when their personal lives are not directly affected by the foreigners at all. However, there is no denying that a wise immigration policy can be beneficial. We need to articulate how immigration serves our economic and societal interests, and have a rational discussion of the pros and cons. It remains to be seen how large-scale immigration can be managed successfully.

The Netherlands has long been hailed as a liberal society with a tolerant immigration policy. However, they underestimated how explosive the situation can become when tolerance gives way to indifference, and a large proportion of the immigrants fail to be integrated into their new communities. Immigration and integration have to go hand in hand. We need an active immigration policy that encourages integration. Newcomers must gradually come to self-identify with their new nation. Immigration policy begins in the country of origin and continues in the host country. It must not be guided by fear, but it has to be taken seriously. Finally, we have to recognize that immigration is essential if we want to preserve our prosperity and our high standard of living.

The discussion about the aging of society should not focus only on the social system and transfer payments, as it is particularly the case in many European countries. This does not do justice to the extent of the change in our society. The question of how increases in life expectancy will change our society requires a far broader discussion.

The first is the question of how society will deal with the increasingly long-lived elderly. Half of all health care spending is already for those over sixty-five. Alzheimer patients can live for many years, but they need constant care. How to care for those suffering from illness, physical or mental weakness is already a difficult challenge. On the one hand, many nurses have low salaries and perform difficult work, while on the other hand there is a growing number of people who need care but cannot afford the necessary round-the-clock expenses. Families are caught between providing care and doing their jobs. How do you finance 24-hour care when it is so labor intensive?

The Japanese currently hold the record in terms of life expectancy. Japan is also a leader in the research and development of robots that one day could help in assisting older people with their day-to-day tasks. In the future, household robots could help compensate for the reduced numbers of working-age population.

The resources required by the elderly are enormous. Already in our discussion about pensions, we considered the burden that underfunded retirement funds place on younger workers. Every time pensions go up, and with each additional retiree, and every year added to our average life expectancy, comes at the expense of the younger ones. These policies are based on the demands of voters, and the younger generation inevitably will fall by the wayside. In this sense, our society must not be just a passive victim of the demographic change but must make a fundamental shift, if we are to avoid tearing ourselves apart in a battle between the generations. A new model of society is needed in which the old must not be seen as playing against the young, but in which there is a shared interest that goes beyond age limits.

This change can only be achieved if a better understanding and awareness of aging can enable us as individuals and as a society to take our future into our hands and to make necessary changes.

All that being said, if the increasing life expectancy is not matched by a longer "health span," we are threatened with the horrifying vision of a morbid society.

"Health span" is that length of time during which we enjoy a reasonably healthy life. The health span is longer if age-related diseases develop later or not at all. We do not know whether some day we will be able to prevent age-related diseases across the board, but we must not leave anything untried. This is the only way to keep our aging society from becoming a society of people with age-related illnesses, with unpredictable consequences.

Large investments will be necessary in biological gerontology research and in the development of preventive therapies, for only a society that consists mainly of spry and mentally alert, strong and capable members will be able to preserve the quality of life of both young and old people.

In order to preserve our society's prosperity, one of the most important transformations will have to take place in the working world. If the average life expectancy reaches well over ninety years, it is inconceivable that the retirement age will have been met more than three decades before.

There will have to be another revolution — a revolution in the division of labor — to follow on the Industrial Revolution of the 19th century. Tasks will have to be broken down differently and tailored to the respective life stages. Continuing education will be seen very differently and become a normal part of the workplace. Physical work will surely have to decrease with age, but mental potentials and abilities must be used in this life period.

This requires a culture of education and training that will enable the human potential to continue developing from youth to old age. Rigid age limits, such as the retirement age, will be a thing of the past. Today one can already see signs of this. We are seeing people who still perform particularly well in old age. Business leaders make decisions in old age. Politicians are able to apply their experience long after the usual age of retirement. Scientists may have new insights many years after "retirement." Productivity can no longer depend solely on young people, but must be shared by young and old alike. This requires that part of our society remains active well into their advanced age.

Reaching the pension should not be the goal of a working life. Anyway, withdrawing suddenly from working life can be fatal, socially and health wise. Rigid retirement at 65, 67 or 70 years often means going into isolation. Compared to the hectic life of the working population, the retiree's endless leisure time seems tempting before you get there, but it is also a bit like being exiled. You are no longer needed. Discrimination against the elderly, however, begins earlier. Even if a thirty-year-old and a seventy-year-old perform almost the same in terms of mental performance, the older person is rarely trusted to learn something new and to do important work.

Age apartheid, however, is poison for a healthy aging society. It is poison for individuals as well. Young people may say that they do not want to live forever but to "fall asleep" after seventy or eighty years; but try to find an eighty-year-old who wants to die tomorrow. Don't be deceived by your own survival instinct. Like all living creatures, humans are programmed for survival, not for dying. But aging also often means suffering from serious diseases. The more positive people are in the face of aging, the higher their life expectancy. It is therefore crucial for our society to understand aging and to develop preventive therapies. Our aging society can only have a future if aging-related diseases can be effectively prevented. This will determine how we evolve as a society as well as coloring the future of every aging individual.

Such preventive therapies will not develop as a matter of course. Scientific progress cannot be planned or predicted. The Industrial Revolution could have taken place two thousand years earlier when the Greek mathematician and engineer Heron of Alexandria invented the steam engine. However, his invention had no practical application in ancient society.

While Europe of the 18th and 19th centuries was *the* engine of innovation, today we are in a phase of consolidation [128]. Anyone born in the middle of the 19th century had a chance to marvel at true technological revolutions, from the invention of the light bulb to the telephone, movies, and cars — these were epochal innovations. Today we feel like we are incredibly advanced when we surf the Internet with a smartphone, but we have hardly figured out what to do with these gadgets beyond confirming our conventional social contacts.

Even China and India are not yet focused on getting ahead by virtue of major inventions and technological advances. Breakthrough innovations are rare indeed. And the pharmaceutical industry prefers to further develop existing medicines rather than struggle to come up with something new.

The process of such "Evergreenings" enables them to renew their patent protection — and thus secure a continuing revenue stream. All they need to do is improve an active substance, even minimally, whereas to develop a new drug is risky and expensive. It is always possible to make a fortune with a "blockbuster" medicine, but drugs that can bring in over a billion dollars in revenue and win this title are rare.

Developing new therapies requires a massive investment. For that reason, the marketing of already patented and approved drugs is much more important to profit-oriented pharmaceutical companies. Small biotechnology companies are more likely to come up with innovations these days. The pharmaceutical sector has largely been consolidated over the past few decades, just like many other industries. Large entities like pharmaceutical giants are never anywhere near as innovative as small companies driven by the entrepreneurial spirit. Developing a drug includes not only finding the active substance and doing preclinical testing, but running clinical trials with the aim of launching the product into the market. The US National Institutes of Health are now developing new drugs and therapies on government contract, taking over some of the classic research for the pharmaceutical industry. As the pharmaceutical companies lose their ability to be innovators, the question arises whether society should take over responsibility for developing new therapies. To make progress, we need to encourage innovation. Where regulation causes an obstacle to therapy development, it should be reviewed.

That being said, new medicines do need to be safe and have the desired therapeutic effect. In addition, new, exclusively marketed drugs are often extremely expensive and are a burden to the public health system and to private payers alike, but pharmaceutical companies need to recover the costs of development, testing and market launch, and they have to show profits. It really does take a major investment to get a new drug ready for clinical trials. First, the tolerability and safety of the drug must be determined in Phase I before the correct dosage is established in Phase II. In Phase III, the success of the therapy has to be proven in thousands of patients, in order to obtain market approval. After approval, Phase IV evaluates the long-term effects of the new drug or treatment over a lengthy period for a greater number of patients.

All these steps are important, because they guarantee the safety of the drugs, whose effectiveness must be clear and well understood. Especially with evidence-based development and testing, modern medicine differs from homeopathy and "traditional" healing procedures for which, paradoxically, some people are willing to spend much more money than for effective medication.

Regulatory hurdles can be obstacles to innovation. This applies first of all to the basic research itself. Each new medication must first be developed in preclinical research and tested on animal models. Concern for animal welfare, which in many countries has now reached a fanatical level, hinders research and innovation. The breeding of animals for human use was a cornerstone for the establishment of civilization ten thousand years ago. Until then, humans had to capture their food base by hunting and gathering, just like many other animal species. Today humans use animals for far more than cattle-raising. Animals, like all living creatures, originally arose from common predecessors, from which they evolved through evolution. Therefore, many of the biological functions in animals are very similar to those of man. Many basic mechanisms can be analyzed by studying simple organisms, such as bacteria, yeast fungi, worms and flies. However, in order to be able to understand a complex organism like human beings, one needs study objects that are closer to us in evolution. Diseases can often be reproduced in mice, but studies on primates are essential for understanding cognition.

Long-term intervention studies of age-related diseases also require models that reproduce human biology as closely as possible. However, until a therapy can be conceptualized at all, it is necessary to have a sufficient understanding of the disease to be treated and the biological processes involved. Diseases and therapies alike affect not only the infected cells and tissues themselves but also have an effect on the entire organism. Neither a disease nor a therapy can be imitated in isolated cells. Many of the interactions in our body are still unknown. That is one reason why results of testing on mammals are so important.

The concept of animal welfare, combined with a deep scientific skepticism, which is mostly fed by ignorance, increases regulatory hurdles and blocks the development of necessary therapies in the long term. Instead of struggling with the bureaucracy, we need an open discussion in which it has to be made clear whether the politically-motivated animal rights activists are ready to do without the healing of the sick in order to save animals from experiments. When you put it in these terms, the extent of this attack on the ethics of our society becomes clearer. The value and dignity of the human being should still take first place.

People sometimes take big health risks out of ignorance. That is precisely why it is indispensable to educate the public and share the high degree of scientific knowledge obtained in the last two hundred years. But we also need every individual to make an effort to participate in the highly praised "knowledge society." Sources of knowledge have never been as freely available as they are today. Meanwhile, knowledge can also be made accessible for the lay audience. Certainly, science journalism has a long way to go to transport knowledge beyond the most highly educated part of society, but it is also up to each individual to ask the right questions and to look for new answers. It is always worthwhile to learn more about ourselves and the world, and the Internet has really made a great contribution here. The critical spirit, however, still lies with the individual herself.

Gerontology researchers are often asked when anti-aging therapy will finally be available. When will research provide those advances that society is paying for? When will age-related diseases be defeated? Billions have been invested in cancer research institutes and dementia centers, but people still die of cancer or lose their memory.

To be able to defeat diseases, one must understand them. The diseases that are associated with aging are highly complex. Pathological changes occur in various tissues in old age. The simpler an organism is, the more dramatic are the successes in life and health prolongation. A mutation in one single gene can double the life of a roundworm. In humans, however, far more complex organs interact and work together. Even cancer is not just a single disease. There are not only different cancer types, but different patients with the same cancer type often need different therapies. We should never commit the error of underestimating the complexity of life. And we can hardly estimate the extent to which human aging will be delayed and whether aging-related diseases can be comprehensively prevented.

But we have our backs to the wall. If we do not find effective means of prevention, the decrepit society we spoke of will become a reality. Health costs will explode, and the ever-aging people will spend years if not decades suffering from disease such as dementia and disability.

However, the epoch-making progress that was achieved just in the last two decades of gerontology research should make us optimistic. If we advance further into the still unknown galaxies of the molecular mechanisms of life and aging, we will be able to extend not only the life span but the "health span" and defeat diseases forever by not letting them arise in the first place.

Since his first written legacies, humankind has been concerned with aging and death, but only modern science has given him insight into his own biological functioning. Scientific progress has led to an enormous increase in knowledge. While biological gerontology research is only a few decades old, it has already gained deep insights into the causes and mechanisms of aging. New approaches to the treatment of age-related diseases are emerging, in regenerative medicine and in preventive measures as well. It is foreseeable that with a consistent pursuit of the gerontology research, old age will no longer be interwoven with suffering and illness but can be marked by vitality. There is a realistic prospect of a good and long life for all.

This demographic change is taking place in almost every human community. People in the 21st century are getting older than ever before — not only in the developed countries of Europe and North America, but also in emerging and developing countries, more and more people are facing a long life. In developing countries, the aging of societies is still offset by their high birth rates, although China, huge as it is, faces the same demographic challenges we do. A healthy aging society is thus not only our own goal but should be the common aspiration of humankind.

Life expectancy keeps rising in most countries in the world even though the widespread obesity has already slowed this trend in the United States. It is unknown whether there is a fixed limit of the longevity humans might achieve. At the Albert Einstein College of Medicine in New York, the Dutch-born gerontologist Jan Vijg recently analyzed the maximum lifespan reached by super centenarians over the past hundred years [129]. He witnessed that until the 1980s the fastest growing age group continuously raised the bar on the age scale and since then leveled off at about 100. The record of super centenarians was set in the late 1990s and has since not been challenged. Based on demographics, there might well be a limit of maximum human lifespan of about 115 years. Time will tell whether medical breakthroughs challenge this in the future. But extending health span is the far more important challenge than purely extending life expectancy further.

So, in conclusion, no — we would not be able to give Gilgamesh the elixir of immortality. Death is as inevitable today as ever. But we could tell Gilgamesh the history of knowledge. We now know why we age and die, even if many mechanisms and connections between aging and disease remain to be clarified.

We are facing great challenges, but never in the history of humanity have we had so many opportunities. It is up to us to seize our chance and to develop ourselves as human beings. A world without disease and suffering is not impossible, but progress is not granted automatically. Advanced cultures can disappear faster than they arose. This applies to ours as well. Only if we keep advancing deeper into thus far unknown worlds, such as the functions of our genes and molecules, we will gain a more complete knowledge of the human being and human aging. We are closer to the understanding of our being today than humanity has been ever before. Taking our destiny in our own hands, should be the goal of our era.

ENDNOTES

[1] N. Sandars, *The Epics of Gilgamesh*. Penguin Books, 2006.

[2] S. L. Miller and H. C. Urey, "Organic compound synthesis on the primitive earth." *Science*, vol. 130, no. 3370, pp. 245–251, Jul. 1959.

[3] A. Hershey and M. Chase, "Independent Functions of Viral Protein and Nucleic Acid in Growth of Bacteriophage," *J Gen Physiol*, vol. 36, no. 1, pp. 39–56, Apr. 1952.

[4] H. F. Judson, *The Eighth Day of Creation*. Cold Spring Harbor Laboratory Press, 1996.

[5] J. D. Watson and F. H. Crick, "Genetical implications of the structure of deoxyribonucleic acid," *Nature*, vol. 171, no. 4361, pp. 964–967, May 1953.

[6] F. Crick, "Central dogma of molecular biology." *Nature*, vol. 227, no. 5258, pp. 561–563, Aug. 1970.

[7] F. H. Crick, L. Barnett, S. Brenner, and R. J. Watts-Tobin, "General nature of the genetic code for proteins," *Nature*, vol. 192, pp. 1227–1232, Dec. 1961.

[8] E. Bianconi, A. Piovesan, F. Facchin, A. Beraudi, R. Casadei, F. Frabetti, L. Vitale, M. C. Pelleri, S. Tassani, F. Piva, S. Perez-Amodio, P. Strippoli, and S. Canaider, "An estimation of the number of cells in the human body." *Ann. Hum. Biol.* vol. 40, no. 6, pp. 463–471, Nov. 2013.

[9] D. A. Sinclair, K. Mills, and L. Guarente, "Accelerated aging and nucleolar fragmentation in yeast sgs1 mutants," *Science*, vol. 277, no. 5330, pp. 1313–1316, Aug. 1997.

[10] H. Aguilaniu, L. Gustafsson, M. Rigoulet, and T. Nyström, "Asymmetric inheritance of oxidatively damaged proteins during cytokinesis." *Science*, vol. 299, no. 5613, pp. 1751–1753, Mar. 2003.

[11] E. J. Stewart, R. Madden, G. Paul, and F. Taddei, "Aging and death in an organism that reproduces by morphologically symmetric division." *PLoS Biol*, vol. 3, no. 2, p. e45, Feb. 2005.

[12] L. Hayflick and P. S. Moorhead, "The serial cultivation of human diploid cell strains," *Exp. Cell Res.* vol. 25, pp. 585–621, Dec. 1961.

[13] P. B. Medawar, "An Unsolved Problem of Biology," *London: Lewis*, 1952.

[14] C. Darwin, *On the Origin of Species*. Penguin UK, 2009.

[15] T. B. Kirkwood and T. Cremer, *Cytogerontology since 1881: a reappraisal of August Weismann and a review of modern progress*, vol. 60, no. 2, pp. 101–121, 1982.

[16] D. Harman, "Aging: a theory based on free radical and radiation chemistry," *J Gerontol*, vol. 11, no. 3, pp. 298–300, Jul. 1956.

[17] S. Brenner, "The genetics of Caenorhabditis elegans," *Genetics*, vol. 77, no. 1, pp. 71–94, Mai 1974.

[18] J. E. Sulston and H. R. Horvitz, "Post-embryonic cell lineages of the nematode, Caenorhabditis elegans," *Developmental biology*, vol. 56, no. 1, pp. 110–156, Mar. 1977.

[19] H. M. Ellis and H. R. Horvitz, "Genetic control of programmed cell death in the nematode C. elegans," *Cell*, vol. 44, no. 6, pp. 817–829, Mar. 1986.

[20] T. E. Johnson, "Increased life-span of age-1 mutants in Caenorhabditis elegans and lower Gompertz rate of aging." *Science*, vol. 249, no. 4971, pp. 908–912, Aug. 1990.

[21] C. Kenyon, J. Chang, E. Gensch, A. Rudner, and R. Tabtiang, "A C. elegans mutant that lives twice as long as wild type." *Nature*, vol. 366, no. 6454, pp. 461–464, Dec. 1993.

[22] D. J. Clancy, D. Gems, L. G. Harshman, S. Oldham, H. Stocker, E. Hafen, S. J. Leevers, and L. Partridge, "Extension of life-span by loss of CHICO, a Drosophila insulin receptor substrate protein," *Science*, vol. 292, no. 5514, pp. 104–106, Apr. 2001.

[23] G. D. Snell, "Dwarf, A New Mendelian Recessive Character of the House Mouse." *Proceedings of the National Academy of Sciences of the United States of America*, vol. 15, no. 9, pp. 733–734, Sep. 1929.

[24] H. Brown-Borg, K. Borg, C. Meliska, and A. Bartke, "Dwarf mice and the ageing process," *Nature*, vol. 384, no. 33, pp. 1–1, Nov. 1996.

[25] M. Holzenberger, J. Dupont, B. Ducos, P. Leneuve, A. Geloen, P. C. Even, P. Cervera, and Y. Le Bouc, "IGF-1 receptor regulates lifespan and resistance

to oxidative stress in mice," *Nature*, vol. 421, no. 6919, pp. 182–187, Jan. 2003.

[26] J. Guevara-Aguirre, P. Balasubramanian, M. Guevara-Aguirre, M. Wei, F. Madia, C. W. Cheng, D. Hwang, A. Martin-Montalvo, J. Saavedra, S. Ingles, R. de Cabo, P. Cohen, and V. D. Longo, "Growth hormone receptor deficiency is associated with a major reduction in pro-aging signaling, cancer, and diabetes in humans," *Sci Transl Med*, vol. 3, no. 70, p. 70ra13, Feb. 2011.

[27] B. J. Willcox, T. A. Donlon, Q. He, R. Chen, J. S. Grove, K. Yano, K. H. Masaki, D. C. Willcox, B. Rodriguez, and J. D. Curb, "FOXO3A genotype is strongly associated with human longevity," *Proceedings of the National Academy of Sciences of the United States of America*, vol. 105, no. 37, pp. 13987–13992, Sep. 2008.

[28] F. Flachsbart, A. Caliebe, R. Kleindorp, H. Blanché, H. von Eller-Eberstein, S. Nikolaus, S. Schreiber, and A. Nebel, "Association of FOXO3A variation with human longevity confirmed in German centenarians." *Proceedings of the National Academy of Sciences of the United States of America*, vol. 106, no. 8, pp. 2700–2705, Feb. 2009.

[29] Y. Suh, G. Atzmon, M. O. Cho, D. Hwang, B. Liu, D. J. Leahy, N. Barzilai, and P. Cohen, "Functionally significant insulin-like growth factor I receptor mutations in centenarians," *Proceedings of the National Academy of Sciences of the United States of America*, vol. 105, no. 9, pp. 3438–3442, Mar. 2008.

[30] J. C. Venter, "The Sequence of the Human Genome," *Science*, vol. 291, no. 5507, pp. 1304–1351, Feb. 2001.

[31] International Human Genome Sequencing Consortium, "Initial sequencing and analysis of the human genome." *Nature*, vol. 409, no. 6822, pp. 860–921, Feb. 2001.

[32] International Human Genome Sequencing Consortium, "Finishing the euchromatic sequence of the human genome." *Nature*, vol. 431, no. 7011, pp. 931–945, Oct. 2004.

[33] M. Eriksson, W. T. Brown, L. B. Gordon, M. W. Glynn, J. Singer, L. Scott, M. R. Erdos, C. M. Robbins, T. Y. Moses, P. Berglund, A. Dutra, E. Pak, S. Durkin, A. B. Csoka, M. Boehnke, T. W. Glover, and F. S. Collins, "Recurrent de novo point mutations in lamin-A cause Hutchinson-Gilford progeria syndrome." *Nature*, vol. 423, no. 6937, pp. 293–298, May 2003.

[34] M. D. Gray, J. C. Shen, A. S. Kamath-Loeb, A. Blank, B. L. Sopher, G. M. Martin, J. Oshima, and L. A. Loeb, "The Werner syndrome protein is a DNA helicase." *Nat. Genet.* vol. 17, no. 1, pp. 100–103, Sep. 1997.

[35] L. H. Hartwell and T. A. Weinert, "Checkpoints: controls that ensure the order of cell cycle events." *Science*, vol. 246, no. 4930, pp. 629–634, Nov. 1989.

[36] M. O. Hengartner, R. E. Ellis, and H. R. Horvitz, "Caenorhabditis elegans gene ced-9 protects cells from programmed cell death," *Nature*, vol. 356, no. 6369, pp. 494–499, Apr. 1992.

[37] M. O. Hengartner and H. R. Horvitz, "C. elegans cell survival gene ced-9 encodes a functional homolog of the mammalian proto-oncogene bcl-2," *Cell*, vol. 76, no. 4, pp. 665–676, Feb. 1994.

[38] B. Maier, W. Gluba, B. Bernier, T. Turner, K. Mohammad, T. Guise, A. Sutherland, M. Thorner, and H. Scrable, "Modulation of mammalian life span by the short isoform of p53," *Genes Dev.* vol. 18, no. 3, pp. 306–319, Feb. 2004.

[39] S. D. Tyner, S. Venkatachalam, J. Choi, S. Jones, N. Ghebranious, H. Igelmann, X. Lu, G. Soron, B. Cooper, C. Brayton, P. S. Hee, T. Thompson, G. Karsenty, A. Bradley, and L. A. Donehower, "p53 mutant mice that display early ageing-associated phenotypes," *Nature*, vol. 415, no. 6867, pp. 45–53, Jan. 2002.

[40] I. Garcia-Cao, M. Garcia-Cao, J. Martin-Caballero, L. M. Criado, P. Klatt, J. M. Flores, J. C. Weill, M. A. Blasco, and M. Serrano, "'Super p53' mice exhibit enhanced DNA damage response, are tumor resistant and age normally," *EMBO J.* vol. 21, no. 22, pp. 6225–6235, Nov. 2002.

[41] A. Matheu, A. Maraver, P. Klatt, I. Flores, I. Garcia-Cao, C. Borras, J. M. Flores, J. Vina, M. A. Blasco, and M. Serrano, "Delayed ageing through damage protection by the Arf/p53 pathway," *Nature*, vol. 448, no. 7151, pp. 375–379, Jul. 2007.

[42] M. O'Driscoll, K. M. Cerosaletti, P. M. Girard, Y. Dai, M. Stumm, B. Kysela, B. Hirsch, A. Gennery, S. E. Palmer, J. Seidel, R. A. Gatti, R. Varon, M. A. Oettinger, H. Neitzel, P. A. Jeggo, and P. Concannon, "DNA ligase IV mutations identified in patients exhibiting developmental delay and immunodeficiency." *Molecular Cell*, vol. 8, no. 6, pp. 1175–1185, Dec. 2001.

[43] J. Cello, A. V. Paul, and E. Wimmer, "Chemical synthesis of poliovirus cDNA: generation of infectious virus in the absence of natural template." *Science*, vol. 297, no. 5583, pp. 1016–1018, Aug. 2002.

[44] D. Hansemann, "Ueber asymmetrische Zelltheilung in Epithelkrebsen und deren biologische Bedeutung," *Archiv f. pathol. Anat.* vol. 119, no. 2, pp. 299–326, Feb. 1890.

[45] T. Boveri, *Zur Frage der Entstehung maligner Tumoren*. Jena: Gustav Fischer, pp. 1–64, 1914.

[46] K. Yamagiwa and K. Ichikawa, "Experimental Study of the Pathogenesis of Carcinoma," vol. 3, pp. 1–29, Jan. 1918.

[47] W. C. Hahn, C. M. Counter, A. S. Lundberg, R. L. Beijersbergen, M. W. Brooks, and R. A. Weinberg, "Creation of human tumour cells with defined genetic elements." *Nature*, vol. 400, no. 6743, pp. 464–468, Jul. 1999.

[48] L. J. Niedernhofer, G. A. Garinis, A. Raams, A. S. Lalai, A. R. Robinson, E. Appeldoorn, H. Odijk, R. Oostendorp, A. Ahmad, W. van Leeuwen, A. F. Theil, W. Vermeulen, G. T. van der Horst, P. Meinecke, W. J. Kleijer, J. Vijg, N. G. Jaspers, and J. H. Hoeijmakers, "A new progeroid syndrome reveals that genotoxic stress suppresses the somatotroph axis," *Nature*, vol. 444, no. 7122, pp. 1038–1043, Dec. 2006.

[49] I. van der Pluijm, G. A. Garinis, R. M. Brandt, T. G. Gorgels, S. W. Wijnhoven, K. E. Diderich, J. de Wit, J. R. Mitchell, C. van Oostrom, R. Beems, L. J. Niedernhofer, S. Velasco, E. C. Friedberg, K. Tanaka, H. van Steeg, J. H. Hoeijmakers, and G. T. van der Horst, "Impaired genome maintenance suppresses the growth hormone–insulin-like growth factor 1 axis in mice with Cockayne syndrome," *PLoS Biol*, vol. 5, no. 1, p. e2, Dec. 2006.

[50] B. Schumacher, I. van der Pluijm, M. J. Moorhouse, T. Kosteas, A. R. Robinson, Y. Suh, T. M. Breit, H. van Steeg, L. J. Niedernhofer, W. van Ijcken, A. Bartke, S. R. Spindler, J. H. J. Hoeijmakers, G. T. J. van der Horst, and G. A. Garinis, "Delayed and accelerated aging share common longevity assurance mechanisms." *PLoS Genet.* vol. 4, no. 8, p. e1000161, Aug. 2008.

[51] G. A. Garinis, L. M. Uittenboogaard, H. Stachelscheid, M. Fousteri, W. van Ijcken, T. M. Breit, H. van Steeg, L. H. F. Mullenders, G. T. J. van der Horst, J. C. Brüning, C. M. Niessen, J. H. J. Hoeijmakers, and B. Schumacher, "Persistent transcription-blocking DNA lesions trigger somatic growth attenuation associated with longevity." *Nat. Cell Biol.* vol. 11, no. 5, pp. 604–615, May 2009.

[52] M. M. Mueller, L. Castells-Roca, V. Babu, M. A. Ermolaeva, R.-U. Müller, P. Frommolt, A. B. Williams, S. Greiss, J. I. Schneider, T. Benzing, B. Schermer, and B. Schumacher, "DAF-16/FOXO and EGL-27/GATA promote developmental growth in response to persistent somatic DNA damage," *Nat. Cell Biol.* vol. 16, no. 12, pp. 1168–1179, Nov. 2014.

[53] G. Mariño, A. P. Ugalde, A. F. Fernández, F. G. Osorio, A. Fueyo, J. M. P. Freije, and C. López-Otín, "Insulin-like growth factor 1 treatment extends longevity in a mouse model of human premature aging by restoring somatotroph axis function." *Proceedings of the National Academy of Sciences of the United States of America*, vol. 107, no. 37, pp. 16268–16273, Sep. 2010.

[54] R. Mostoslavsky, K. F. Chua, D. B. Lombard, W. W. Pang, M. R. Fischer, L. Gellon, P. Liu, G. Mostoslavsky, S. Franco, M. M. Murphy, K. D. Mills, P. Patel, J. T. Hsu, A. L. Hong, E. Ford, H. L. Cheng, C. Kennedy, N. Nunez, R. Bronson, D. Frendewey, W. Auerbach, D. Valenzuela, M. Karow, M. O.

Hottiger, S. Hursting, J. C. Barrett, L. Guarente, R. Mulligan, B. Demple, G. D. Yancopoulos, and F. W. Alt, "Genomic instability and aging-like phenotype in the absence of mammalian SIRT6," *Cell*, vol. 124, no. 2, pp. 315–329, Jan. 2006.

[55] Z. Song, J. Wang, L. M. Guachalla, G. Terszowski, H. R. Rodewald, Z. Ju, and K. L. Rudolph, "Alterations of the systemic environment are the primary cause of impaired B and T lymphopoiesis in telomere-dysfunctional mice," *Blood*, vol. 115, no. 8, pp. 1481–1489, Feb. 2010.

[56] A. Alzheimer, "*Uber eine eigenartige Erkrankung der Hirnrinde.*" *Allg. Z. Psychiat. Psych.-Gerichtl. Med.* vol. 64, no. 1, pp. 146–148, Mar. 1907.

[57] U. Müller, P. Winter, and M. B. Graeber, "A presenilin 1 mutation in the first case of Alzheimer's disease." *Lancet Neurol*, vol. 12, no. 2, pp. 129–130, Feb. 2013.

[58] E. H. Corder, A. M. Saunders, W. J. Strittmatter, D. E. Schmechel, P. C. Gaskell, G. W. Small, A. D. Roses, J. L. Haines, and M. A. Pericak-Vance, "Gene dose of apolipoprotein E type 4 allele and the risk of Alzheimer's disease in late onset families." *Science*, vol. 261, no. 5123, pp. 921–923, Aug. 1993.

[59] W. J. Strittmatter, A. M. Saunders, D. Schmechel, M. Pericak-Vance, J. Enghild, G. S. Salvesen, and A. D. Roses, "Apolipoprotein E: high-avidity binding to beta-amyloid and increased frequency of type 4 allele in late-onset familial Alzheimer disease." *Proceedings of the National Academy of Sciences of the United States of America*, vol. 90, no. 5, pp. 1977–1981, Mar. 1993.

[60] C.-C. Liu, T. Kanekiyo, H. Xu, and G. Bu, "Apolipoprotein E and Alzheimer disease: risk, mechanisms and therapy," *Nat Rev Neurol*, vol. 9, no. 2, pp. 106–118, Jan. 2013.

[61] P. Syntichaki, K. Troulinaki, and N. Tavernarakis, "eIF4E function in somatic cells modulates ageing in Caenorhabditis elegans," *Nature*, vol. 445, no. 7130, pp. 922–926, Feb. 2007.

[62] G. Angelo and M. R. Van Gilst, "Starvation protects germline stem cells and extends reproductive longevity in C. elegans." *Science*, vol. 326, no. 5955, pp. 954–958, Nov. 2009.

[63] N. A. Bishop and L. Guarente, "Two neurons mediate diet-restriction-induced longevity in C. elegans," *Nature*, vol. 447, no. 7144, pp. 545–549, May 2007.

[64] C. Kang and L. Avery, "Systemic regulation of starvation response in Caenorhabditis elegans." *Genes Dev.* vol. 23, no. 1, pp. 12–17, Jan. 2009.

[65] R. C. Grandison, M. D. W. Piper, and L. Partridge, "Amino-acid imbalance explains extension of lifespan by dietary restriction in Drosophila." *Nature*, vol. 462, no. 7276, pp. 1061–1064, Dec. 2009.

[66] R. J. Colman, R. M. Anderson, S. C. Johnson, E. K. Kastman, K. J. Kosmatka, T. M. Beasley, D. B. Allison, C. Cruzen, H. A. Simmons, J. W. Kemnitz, and R. Weindruch, "Caloric restriction delays disease onset and mortality in rhesus monkeys," *Science*, vol. 325, no. 5937, pp. 201–204, Jul. 2009.

[67] J. A. Mattison, G. S. Roth, T. M. Beasley, E. M. Tilmont, A. M. Handy, R. L. Herbert, D. L. Longo, D. B. Allison, J. E. Young, M. Bryant, D. Barnard, W. F. Ward, W. Qi, D. K. Ingram, and R. de Cabo, "Impact of caloric restriction on health and survival in rhesus monkeys from the NIA study." *Nature*, vol. 489, no. 7415, pp. 318–321, Sep. 2012.

[68] M. C. Vogt, L. Paeger, S. Hess, S. M. Steculorum, M. Awazawa, B. Hampel, S. Neupert, H. T. Nicholls, J. Mauer, A. C. Hausen, R. Predel, P. Kloppenburg, T. L. Horvath, and J. C. Brüning, "Neonatal insulin action impairs hypothalamic neurocircuit formation in response to maternal high-fat feeding." *Cell*, vol. 156, no. 3, pp. 495–509, Jan. 2014.

[69] D. E. Harrison, R. Strong, Z. D. Sharp, J. F. Nelson, C. M. Astle, K. Flurkey, N. L. Nadon, J. E. Wilkinson, K. Frenkel, C. S. Carter, M. Pahor, M. A. Javors, E. Fernandez, and R. A. Miller, "Rapamycin fed late in life extends lifespan in genetically heterogeneous mice," *Nature*, vol. 460, no. 7253, pp. 392-395, Jul. 2009.

[70] P. Mitchell, "Coupling of phosphorylation to electron and hydrogen transfer by a chemi-osmotic type of mechanism." *Nature*, vol. 191, pp. 144–148, Jul. 1961.

[71] T. L. Parkes, A. J. Elia, D. Dickinson, A. J. Hilliker, J. P. Phillips, and G. L. Boulianne, "Extension of Drosophila lifespan by overexpression of human SOD1 in motorneurons." *Nat. Genet.* vol. 19, no. 2, pp. 171–174, Jun. 1998.

[72] J. P. Phillips, S. D. Campbell, D. Michaud, M. Charbonneau, and A. J. Hilliker, "Null mutation of copper/zinc superoxide dismutase in Drosophila confers hypersensitivity to paraquat and reduced longevity." *Proceedings of the National Academy of Sciences of the United States of America*, vol. 86, no. 8, pp. 2761–2765, Apr. 1989.

[73] R. Doonan, J. J. McElwee, F. Matthijssens, G. A. Walker, K. Houthoofd, P. Back, A. Matscheski, J. R. Vanfleteren, and D. Gems, "Against the oxidative damage theory of aging: superoxide dismutases protect against oxidative stress but have little or no effect on life span in Caenorhabditis elegans," *Genes Dev.* vol. 22, no. 23, pp. 3236–3241, Dec. 2008.

[74] V. I. Pérez, H. Van Remmen, A. Bokov, C. J. Epstein, J. Vijg, and A. Richardson, "The overexpression of major antioxidant enzymes does not extend the lifespan of mice." *Aging Cell*, vol. 8, no. 1, pp. 73–75, Feb. 2009.

[75] S. E. Schriner, N. J. Linford, G. M. Martin, P. Treuting, C. E. Ogburn, M. Emond, P. E. Coskun, W. Ladiges, N. Wolf, H. Van Remmen, D. C. Wallace, and P. S. Rabinovitch, "Extension of murine life span by overexpression

of catalase targeted to mitochondria." *Science*, vol. 308, no. 5730, pp. 1909–1911, Jun. 2005.

[76] M. G. Spillantini, M. L. Schmidt, V. M. Lee, J. Q. Trojanowski, R. Jakes, and M. Goedert, "Alpha-synuclein in Lewy bodies." *Nature*, vol. 388, no. 6645, pp. 839–840, Aug. 1997.

[77] A. Ameur, J. B. Stewart, C. Freyer, E. Hagstrom, M. Ingman, N. G. Larsson, and U. Gyllensten, "Ultra-deep sequencing of mouse mitochondrial DNA: mutational patterns and their origins," *PLoS Genet.* vol. 7, no. 3, p. e1002028, Mar. 2011.

[78] A. Trifunovic, A. Wredenberg, M. Falkenberg, J. N. Spelbrink, A. T. Rovio, C. E. Bruder, Y. Bohlooly, S. Gidlof, A. Oldfors, R. Wibom, J. Tornell, H. T. Jacobs, and N. G. Larsson, "Premature ageing in mice expressing defective mitochondrial DNA polymerase," *Nature*, vol. 429, no. 6990, pp. 417–423, May 2004.

[79] J. M. Ross, J. B. Stewart, E. Hagström, S. Brené, A. Mourier, G. Coppotelli, C. Freyer, M. Lagouge, B. J. Hoffer, L. Olson, and N.-G. Larsson, "Germline mitochondrial DNA mutations aggravate ageing and can impair brain development." *Nature*, vol. 501, no. 7467, pp. 412-4155, Sep. 2013.

[80] C. W. Greider and E. H. Blackburn, "Identification of a specific telomere terminal transferase activity in Tetrahymena extracts." *Cell*, vol. 43, no. 2, pp. 405–413, Dec. 1985.

[81] M. Jaskelioff, F. L. Muller, J. H. Paik, E. Thomas, S. Jiang, A. C. Adams, E. Sahin, M. Kost-Alimova, A. Protopopov, J. Cadinanos, J. W. Horner, E. Maratos-Flier, and R. A. DePinho, "Telomerase reactivation reverses tissue degeneration in aged telomerase-deficient mice," *Nature*, vol. 469, no. 7328, pp. 102–106, Jan. 2011.

[82] D. J. Baker, K. B. Jeganathan, J. D. Cameron, M. Thompson, S. Juneja, A. Kopecka, R. Kumar, R. B. Jenkins, de Groen, P. C. P. Roche, and J. M. van Deursen, "BubR1 insufficiency causes early onset of aging-associated phenotypes and infertility in mice," *Nat. Genet.* vol. 36, no. 7, pp. 744–749, Jul. 2004.

[83] A. R. Choudhury, Z. Ju, M. W. Djojosubroto, A. Schienke, A. Lechel, S. Schaetzlein, H. Jiang, A. Stepczynska, C. Wang, J. Buer, H. W. Lee, T. Von Zglinicki, A. Ganser, P. Schirmacher, H. Nakauchi, and K. L. Rudolph, "Cdkn1a deletion improves stem cell function and lifespan of mice with dysfunctional telomeres without accelerating cancer formation," *Nat. Genet.* vol. 39, no. 1, pp. 99–105, Jan. 2007.

[84] D. J. Baker, T. Wijshake, T. Tchkonia, N. K. LeBrasseur, B. G. Childs, B. van de Sluis, J. L. Kirkland, and J. M. van Deursen, "Clearance of p16Ink4a-positive senescent cells delays ageing-associated disorders," *Nature*, vol. 479, no. 7372, pp. 232-236, Nov. 2011.

[85] R. M. Cawthon, K. R. Smith, E. O'Brien, A. Sivatchenko, and R. A. Kerber, "Association between telomere length in blood and mortality in people aged 60 years or older." *Lancet*, vol. 361, no. 9355, pp. 393–395, Feb. 2003.

[86] D. Muñoz-Espín, M. Cañamero, A. Maraver, G. Gómez-López, J. Contreras, S. Murillo-Cuesta, A. Rodríguez-Baeza, I. Varela-Nieto, J. Ruberte, M. Collado, and M. Serrano, "Programmed Cell Senesceduring Mammalian Embryonic Development," *Cell*, vol. 155, no. 5, pp. 1104–1118, Nov. 2013.

[87] Y. Hong, R. Roy, and V. Ambros, "Developmental regulation of a cyclin-dependent kinase inhibitor controls postembryonic cell cycle progression in Caenorhabditis elegans," *Development*, vol. 125, no. 18, pp. 3585–3597, 9/1998 1998. M. Storer, A. Mas, A. Robert-Moreno, M. Pecoraro, M. C. Ortells, V. Di Giacomo, R. Yosef, N. Pilpel, V. Krizhanovsky, J. Sharpe, and W. M. Keyes, "Senescence is a developmental mechanism that contributes to embryonic growth and patterning." *Cell*, vol. 155, no. 5, pp. 1119–1130, Nov. 2013.

[88] S. Parrinello, E. Samper, A. Krtolica, J. Goldstein, S. Melov, and J. Campisi, "Oxygen sensitivity severely limits the replicative lifespan of murine fibroblasts," *Nat. Cell Biol.* vol. 5, no. 8, pp. 741–747, Aug. 2003.

[89] A. Krtolica, S. Parrinello, S. Lockett, P. Y. Desprez, and J. Campisi, "Senescent fibroblasts promote epithelial cell growth and tumorigenesis: a link between cancer and aging." *Proceedings of the National Academy of Sciences of the United States of America*, vol. 98, no. 21, pp. 12072–12077, Oct. 2001.

[90] F. Rodier, J. P. Coppe, C. K. Patil, W. A. Hoeijmakers, D. P. Munoz, S. R. Raza, A. Freund, E. Campeau, A. R. Davalos, and J. Campisi, "Persistent DNA damage signalling triggers senescence-associated inflammatory cytokine secretion," *Nat. Cell Biol.* vol. 11, no. 8, pp. 973–979, Aug. 2009.

[91] C. P. Martins, L. Brown-Swigart, and G. I. Evan, "Modeling the therapeutic efficacy of p53 restoration in tumors." *Cell*, vol. 127, no. 7, pp. 1323–1334, Dec. 2006.

[92] W. Xue, L. Zender, C. Miething, R. A. Dickins, E. Hernando, V. Krizhanovsky, C. Cordon-Cardo, and S. W. Lowe, "Senescence and tumour clearance is triggered by p53 restoration in murine liver carcinomas," *Nature*, vol. 445, no. 7128, pp. 656–660, Feb. 2007.

[93] I. M. Toller, K. J. Neelsen, M. Steger, M. L. Hartung, M. O. Hottiger, M. Stucki, B. Kalali, M. Gerhard, A. A. Sartori, M. Lopes, and A. Muller, "Carcinogenic bacterial pathogen Helicobacter pylori triggers DNA double-strand breaks and a DNA damage response in its host cells," *Proceedings of the National Academy of Sciences of the United States of America*, vol. 108, no. 36, pp. 14944–14949, Sep. 2011.

[94] F. G. Osorio, C. Bárcena, C. Soria-Valles, A. J. Ramsay, F. de Carlos, J. Cobo, A. Fueyo, J. M. P. Freije, and C. López-Otín, "Nuclear lamina defects cause ATM-dependent NF-kB activation and link accelerated aging to a systemic inflammatory response." *Genes & development*, vol. 26, no. 20, pp. 2311–2324, Oct. 2012.

[95] J. S. Tilstra, A. R. Robinson, J. Wang, S. Q. Gregg, C. L. Clauson, D. P. Reay, L. A. Nasto, C. M. St Croix, A. Usas, N. Vo, J. Huard, P. R. Clemens, D. B. Stolz, D. C. Guttridge, S. C. Watkins, G. A. Garinis, Y. Wang, L. J. Niedernhofer, and P. D. Robbins, "NF-B inhibition delays DNA damage-induced senescence and aging in mice." *J. Clin. Invest.* vol. 122, no. 7, pp. 2601–2612, Jul. 2012.

[96] M. A. Ermolaeva, A. Segref, A. Dakhovnik, H.-L. Ou, J. I. Schneider, O. Utermöhlen, T. Hoppe, and B. Schumacher, "DNA damage in germ cells induces an innate immune response that triggers systemic stress resistance." *Nature*, vol. 501, no. 7467, pp. 416–420, Sep. 2013.

[97] J. Karpac, A. Younger, and H. Jasper, "Dynamic coordination of innate immune signaling and insulin signaling regulates systemic responses to localized DNA damage," *Dev. Cell*, vol. 20, no. 6, pp. 841–854, Jun. 2011.

[98] H. Jiang, P. H. Patel, A. Kohlmaier, M. O. Grenley, D. G. McEwen, and B. A. Edgar, "Cytokine/Jak/Stat signaling mediates regeneration and homeostasis in the Drosophila midgut." *Cell*, vol. 137, no. 7, pp. 1343–1355, Jun. 2009.

[99] H. Hsin and C. Kenyon, "Signals from the reproductive system regulate the lifespan of C. elegans." *Nature*, vol. 399, no. 6734, pp. 362–366, May 1999.

[100] S. L. Cargill, J. R. Carey, H.-G. Müller, and G. Anderson, "Age of ovary determines remaining life expectancy in old ovariectomized mice." *Aging Cell*, vol. 2, no. 3, pp. 185–190, Jun. 2003.

[101] J. B. Hamilton and G. E. Mestler, "Mortality and survival: comparison of eunuchs with intact men and women in a mentally retarded population." *J Gerontol*, vol. 24, no. 4, pp. 395–411, Oct. 1969.

[102] K.-J. Min, C.-K. Lee, and H.-N. Park, "The lifespan of Korean eunuchs." *Curr. Biol.* vol. 22, no. 18, pp. R792–3, Sep. 2012.

[103] E. C. Berg and A. A. Maklakov, "Sexes suffer from suboptimal lifespan because of genetic conflict in a seed beetle." *Proc. Biol. Sci.* vol. 279, no. 1745, pp. 4296–4302, Oct. 2012.

[104] M. Lahdenperä, V. Lummaa, S. Helle, M. Tremblay, and A. F. Russell, "Fitness benefits of prolonged post-reproductive lifespan in women." *Nature*, vol. 428, no. 6979, pp. 178–181, Mar. 2004.

[105] H. Schulz, "Ueber Hefegifte," *Pflugers Arch. Ges. Physiol.* vol. 42, pp. 517–541, 1888.

[106] C. M. Southam and J. Ehrlich, "Effects of extract of western red-cedar heartwood on certain wood-decaying fungi in culture." *Phytopathology*, vol. 33, pp. 517–524, 1943.

[107] E. J. Calabrese, "Hormesis and medicine," *Br J Clin Pharmacol*, vol. 66, no. 5, pp. 594–617, Nov. 2008.

[108] D. Susa, J. R. Mitchell, M. Verweij, M. van de Ven, H. Roest, S. van den Engel, I. Bajema, K. Mangundap, J. N. Ijzermans, J. H. Hoeijmakers, and R. W. de Bruin, "Congenital DNA repair deficiency results in protection against renal ischemia reperfusion injury in mice," *Aging Cell*, vol. 8, no. 2, pp. 192–200, Apr. 2009.

[109] M. Ristow, K. Zarse, A. Oberbach, N. Klöting, M. Birringer, M. Kiehntopf, M. Stumvoll, C. R. Kahn, and M. Blüher, "Antioxidants prevent health-promoting effects of physical exercise in humans." *Proceedings of the National Academy of Sciences of the United States of America*, vol. 106, no. 21, pp. 8665–8670, May 2009.

[110] J. Jans, W. Schul, Y. G. Sert, Y. Rijksen, H. Rebel, A. P. Eker, S. Nakajima, H. van Steeg, F. R. de Gruijl, A. Yasui, J. H. Hoeijmakers, and G. T. van der Horst, "Powerful skin cancer protection by a CPD-photolyase transgene," *Curr. Biol.* vol. 15, no. 2, pp. 105–115, Jan. 2005.

[111] T. Eisenberg, H. Knauer, A. Schauer, S. Büttner, C. Ruckenstuhl, D. Carmona-Gutierrez, J. Ring, S. Schroeder, C. Magnes, L. Antonacci, H. Fussi, L. Deszcz, R. Hartl, E. Schraml, A. Criollo, E. Megalou, D. Weiskopf, P. Laun, G. Heeren, M. Breitenbach, B. Grubeck-Loebenstein, E. Herker, B. Fahrenkrog, K.-U. Fröhlich, F. Sinner, N. Tavernarakis, N. Minois, G. Kroemer, and F. Madeo, "Induction of autophagy by spermidine promotes longevity," *Nat. Cell Biol.* vol. 11, no. 11, pp. 1305–1314, Nov. 2009.

[112] V. K. Gupta, L. Scheunemann, T. Eisenberg, S. Mertel, A. Bhukel, T. S. Koemans, J. M. Kramer, K. S. Y. Liu, S. Schroeder, H. G. Stunnenberg, F. Sinner, C. Magnes, T. R. Pieber, S. Dipt, A. Fiala, A. Schenck, M. Schwaerzel, F. Madeo, and S. J. Sigrist, "Restoring polyamines protects from age-induced memory impairment in an autophagy-dependent manner." *Nat. Neurosci.* vol. 16, no. 10, pp. 1453–1460, Oct. 2013.

[113] E. Cohen, J. F. Paulsson, P. Blinder, T. Burstyn-Cohen, D. Du, G. Estepa, A. Adame, H. M. Pham, M. Holzenberger, J. W. Kelly, E. Masliah, and A. Dillin, "Reduced IGF-1 signaling delays age-associated proteotoxicity in mice." *Cell*, vol. 139, no. 6, pp. 1157–1169, Dec. 2009.

[114] S. Freude, M. M. Hettich, C. Schumann, O. Stöhr, L. Koch, C. Köhler, M. Udelhoven, U. Leeser, M. Müller, N. Kubota, T. Kadowaki, W. Krone, H. Schröder, J. C. Brüning, and M. Schubert, "Neuronal IGF-1 resistance reduces Abeta accumulation and protects against premature death in a model of Alzheimer's disease." *FASEB J.* vol. 23, no. 10, pp. 3315–3324, Oct. 2009.

[115] G. de Haan, W. Nijhof, and G. Van Zant, "Mouse strain-dependent changes in frequency and proliferation of hematopoietic stem cells during aging: correlation between lifespan and cycling activity." *Blood*, vol. 89, no. 5, pp. 1543–1550, Mar. 1997.

[116] I. M. Conboy, M. J. Conboy, A. J. Wagers, E. R. Girma, I. L. Weissman, and T. A. Rando, "Rejuvenation of aged progenitor cells by exposure to a young systemic environment." *Nature*, vol. 433, no. 7027, pp. 760–764, Feb. 2005.

[117] M. Sinha, Y. C. Jang, J. Oh, D. Khong, E. Y. Wu, R. Manohar, C. Miller, S. G. Regalado, F. S. Loffredo, J. R. Pancoast, M. F. Hirshman, J. Lebowitz, J. L. Shadrach, M. Cerletti, M.-J. Kim, T. Serwold, L. J. Goodyear, B. Rosner, R. T. Lee, and A. J. Wagers, "Restoring Systemic GDF11 Levels Reverses Age-Related Dysfunction in Mouse Skeletal Muscle." *Science*, vol. 344, no. 6184, pp. 649-652, May 2014.

[118] J. B. Gurdon, T. R. Elsdale, and M. Fischberg, "Sexually mature individuals of Xenopus laevis from the transplantation of single somatic nuclei." *Nature*, vol. 182, no. 4627, pp. 64–65, Jul. 1958.

[119] K. Takahashi and S. Yamanaka, "Induction of pluripotent stem cells from mouse embryonic and adult fibroblast cultures by defined factors." *Cell*, vol. 126, no. 4, pp. 663–676, Aug. 2006.

[120] K. Takahashi, K. Tanabe, M. Ohnuki, M. Narita, T. Ichisaka, K. Tomoda, and S. Yamanaka, "Induction of pluripotent stem cells from adult human fibroblasts by defined factors." *Cell*, vol. 131, no. 5, pp. 861–872, Nov. 2007.

[121] B. Rogina, S. L. Helfand, and S. Frankel, "Longevity regulation by Drosophila Rpd3 deacetylase and caloric restriction." *Science*, vol. 298, no. 5599, p. 1745, Nov. 2002.

[122] H. A. Tissenbaum and L. Guarente, "Increased dosage of a sir-2 gene extends lifespan in Caenorhabditis elegans," *Nature*, vol. 410, no. 6825, pp. 227–230, Mar. 2001.

[123] K. T. Howitz, K. J. Bitterman, H. Y. Cohen, D. W. Lamming, S. Lavu, J. G. Wood, R. E. Zipkin, P. Chung, A. Kisielewski, L. L. Zhang, B. Scherer, and D. A. Sinclair, "Small molecule activators of sirtuins extend Saccharomyces cerevisiae lifespan," *Nature*, vol. 425, no. 6954, pp. 191–196, Sep. 2003.

[124] J. A. Baur, K. J. Pearson, N. L. Price, H. A. Jamieson, C. Lerin, A. Kalra, V. V. Prabhu, J. S. Allard, G. Lopez-Lluch, K. Lewis, P. J. Pistell, S. Poosala, K. G. Becker, O. Boss, D. Gwinn, M. Wang, S. Ramaswamy, K. W. Fishbein, R. G. Spencer, E. G. Lakatta, D. Le Couteur, R. J. Shaw, P. Navas, P. Puigserver, D. K. Ingram, R. de Cabo, and D. A. Sinclair, "Resveratrol improves health and survival of mice on a high-calorie diet," *Nature*, vol. 444, no. 7117, pp. 337–342, Nov. 2006.

[125] M. Pacholec, J. E. Bleasdale, B. Chrunyk, D. Cunningham, D. Flynn, R. S. Garofalo, D. Griffith, M. Griffor, P. Loulakis, B. Pabst, X. Qiu, B. Stockman, V. Thanabal, A. Varghese, J. Ward, J. Withka, and K. Ahn, "SRT1720, SRT2183, SRT1460, and Resveratrol Are Not Direct Activators of SIRT1," *J Biol Chem*, vol. 285, no. 11, pp. 8340–8351, Mar. 2010.

[126] D. Beher, J. Wu, S. Cumine, K. W. Kim, S.-C. Lu, L. Atangan, and M. Wang, "Resveratrol is Not a Direct Activator of SIRT1 Enzyme Activity," *Chemical Biology & Drug Design*, vol. 74, no. 6, pp. 619–624, Dec. 2009.

[127] C. Burnett, S. Valentini, F. Cabreiro, M. Goss, M. Somogyvári, M. D. Piper, M. Hoddinott, G. L. Sutphin, V. Leko, J. J. McElwee, R. P. Vázquez-Manrique, A.-M. Orfila, D. Ackerman, C. Au, G. Vinti, M. Riesen, K. Howard, C. Neri, A. Bedalov, M. Kaeberlein, C. Soti, L. Partridge, and D. Gems, "Absence of effects of Sir2 overexpression on lifespan in C. elegans and Drosophila." *Nature*, vol. 477, no. 7365, pp. 482–485, Sep. 2011.

[128] J. Vijg, *The American Technological Challenge*. Algora Publishing, 2011.

[129] X. Dong, B. Milholland, J. Vijg, "Evidence for a limit to human lifespan," *Nature*, vol. 538, no. 7624, pp. 257-259, Oct. 2016

INDEX

Printed in the United States
By Bookmasters